Bekindr

The Transformative Power of Kindness

Eva Ritvo, MD

MOMOSA PUBLISHING

Printed in the United States of America.
Cover art: Anthony Liggins
Cover design: Lorena Fernandez
Interior design: Martin Rouillard

Library of Congress Number 2017915477.
ISBN 978-0-9994151-0-8
2 4 6 8 10 9 7 5 3 hardcover
Visit our parent company at MomosaPublishing.com

*To my daughters, Joy and Gigi
and my kind stranger, Louie*

TABLE OF CONTENTS

"To be doing good deeds is man's most glorious task."

—*Sophocles*

Introduction

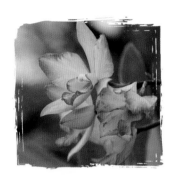

Welcome! You just picked up (or downloaded) a book on kindness! And that's a great first step in the process of making our world just a bit better.

This book invites you into the lives of others to see how kindness has impacted them. Sixty-four contributors share their stories in their own words. Woven between these narratives, I bring you facts, figures and quotes about kindness to support your journey to Bekindr. Most likely, I am "preaching to the choir," but I hope you will find meaning and be moved to share what you learn with others.

I would like to set the stage with some background from the social and health sciences and let you know how *Bekindr* was founded. But feel free to dive right into the first story if that is your preference.

"Teach this triple truth to all: A generous heart, kind speech, and a life of service and compassion are things which renew humanity."

—Buddha

Did you know we are living in the most peaceful time in human history? Although the twenty-four-hour news cycle would have us think otherwise, the data support this optimistic view of our era. In his bestseller, *Better Angels of Our Nature*, Harvard psychologist Steven Pinker shows that Darwin was right when he predicted that our inborn desire to help others is a powerful driver of human evolution. In the words of psychologist Stefan Klein, it's "survival of the nicest."

Did you know that children by the age of fourteen months old exhibit kindness? Dr. Michael Tomasello at the Max Planck Institute has observed that when babies see an adult with full hands struggling to open a door, they try to help. Each of us is born with an innate propensity to aid others, a drive that can be nurtured or extinguished over time.

Can kindness make you happier? Dr. Sonja Lyubomirsky, at the University of California, Riverside, along with her colleagues, assigned students to perform five random acts of kindness a week. Six weeks later, at the end of the study, the students who performed all five acts, on the same day, had significantly increased their levels of happiness.

Is kindness contagious? Yes! Simply watching a video of Mother Teresa for ten minutes made viewers feel better and subsequently behave in a kinder fashion. Dr. Jonathan Haidt, at New York University Stern School of Business, designed the study and calls the phenomenon he observed "elevation." He says, elevation "is an emotional response to moral beauty" that "makes an individual feel lifted up and optimistic about humanity." When we see an act of kindness, we get a warm feeling in our chests and are inspired to act in a kinder way.

We have cells in our brains that fire when we act and when we see an action performed. Scientists in Parma, Italy first discovered these special neurons in the 1990s when they were studying the function of different brain regions in monkeys. The scientists took a snack break, and they noticed that the monkey's brain lit up (fired) in the motor cortex region responsible for tongue movement when the monkey saw the scientists eating. They aptly named these cells "mirror neurons" and they go a long way toward explaining our feelings and behaviors.

Mirror neurons, for instance, explain why it's easier to exercise in groups, why athletes spend so much time watching other athletes, why we are drawn to happy people, and why kindness is contagious. "When you smile, the whole world smiles with you," now has a scientific explanation. It works the other way too, so when you come home in a bad mood and wonder why your spouse/child/roommate seems irritable, look no further than his/her mirror neurons to understand why.

So, if you want to Bekindr, simply surround yourself with people, shows and stories about kindness, and your brain will respond in kind—pun intended!

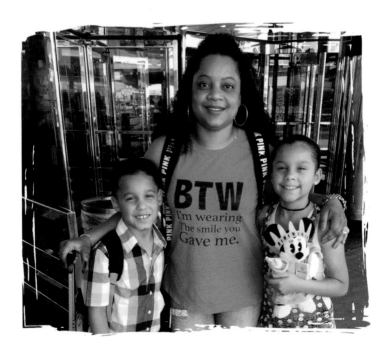

The warm feeling in our chests that Dr. Haidt observed most likely comes from a substance called oxytocin. Scientists have nicknamed oxytocin the "love" or "cuddle hormone." It is released in a variety of circumstances including childbirth, nursing and physical intimacy. Hugging, warm showers, baths and laughter all trigger the release of oxytocin. Oxytocin helps us feel connected, increases trust and raises our desire to help others. It not only makes us feel better, but it also improves our physical health by decreasing levels of the stress hormone cortisol as well as inflammation throughout the body.

According to Eva Selhub, MD in *The Love Response*, kindness also helps us control our heart rate. Research shows that thinking, praying or meditating about kindness for ten minutes a day for two months will increase your vagal tone and slow your heart rate. Vagal tone is the degree of activity occurring within the parasympathetic nervous system, responsible for our "rest and digest" response; it counteracts our sympathetic nervous system responsible for our "fight or flight" response. Enhancing your vagal tone helps you lower your resting heart rate. We feel calmer when our heart is beating at a lower rate. By learning to slow your heart, you can improve your mental and physical health. When we exhale, our vagus nerve is activated and our heart rate slows. So when you feel upset, remember to take a deep breath and let it all the way out. And when you have a chance to give, receive or even observe kindness, grab it!

In *Survival of the Nicest*, Stefan Klein writes: "The history of humankind began with an altruistic revolution—our ancestors started to care for their fellows." These ancestors lived in small groups of 100–150 people, all of whom they knew intimately. Everyone's survival was tied to the group. As our brains evolved, so did our ability to cooperate and care for one another. Scientists hypothesize that dramatic changes in human behavior occurred around 100,000 years ago and were possibly brought about by a rapid expansion of the portion of our brain containing mirror neurons. This growth allowed our predecessors to feel more empathy for one another and to learn more quickly by imitation thus giving rise to civilization as we know it.

Over time, our group of "fellows" has widened. Print, radio and telephones radically altered the number of people with whom we interact. Social connections broadened as travel became easier and easier. Then the advent of the Internet created the most sweeping changes yet. Our social circles have expanded exponentially. We can now interact with hundreds of thousands of people scattered around the globe in a matter of minutes. Messages, videos and GIFs now "go viral," meaning that people are experiencing the same thing around the world almost simultaneously.

Such rapid change in our social structure has certainly caused some growing pains. With progress comes regression. We are seeing both. Of course, it is difficult to embrace all of humanity. But if we are to live in such an interconnected world, our brains must learn to adapt. Our inborn suspicion of diversity must be overcome and replaced with a more modern understanding that we are more alike than different, and that we are all here experiencing the human condition together. We must continue to empathize with one another and learn from one another, as our brains are designed to do. We must continue to support one another even under the strain of so many social connections.

Kindness requires effort. We must understand the needs of others and take time to figure out how to help. The more complex the problem, the more time is required to assist. It is easier to help someone you know well because you are better able to understand his or her needs. Thus, while it is natural to feel most comfortable in groups of people with similar experiences and needs, we must continue to grow and evolve and learn to care for more of our fellow human beings, including those with diverse backgrounds, cultures, and life experiences.

In 2015, with the assistance of friends and colleagues Craig Calvert and Adeline Oka and my daughter Joy, I founded Bekindr to create a place to gather and share stories of being positively impacted by others. Since its inception, we have received hundreds of uplifting stories, many of which you will read in this book. Stories teach and inspire us to become the best versions of ourselves, and I hope you will find that to be the case as you read on.

As we learn about others, we become less fearful of them. Expanded exposure allows us to grow to understand that we are all indeed a family. Our survival and well-being depend on helping one another.

We need kindness when we are in trouble or distress. Our vulnerability often motivates us to connect with others. Dr. Brené Brown, in her popular TED talk, entitled "The Power of Vulnerability," eloquently describes the gift that comes when we acknowledge our own needs and let someone in to help.

I am deeply grateful to everyone who shared their story. For many, it wasn't easy to recall these moments. It was often difficult to read or hear about these struggles. As a reader, you might find some of the stories upsetting. The goal is to help you incorporate more kindness and hope into your world, not to distress you. So, if you can hang in there and finish the story, you will see that kindness helped heal even the deepest of wounds or lighten even the heaviest of burdens. If you find particular stories too troubling, skip over them. There is plenty to be learned without reading every word. Please remember that all contributors took a risk when they chose to share their story, and I hope you will offer them compassion and kindness in return.

I once heard it said that life is like a string of pearls: there are lots of knots in between the moments that we treasure. Through acts of kindness, which we extend to others, receive or even witness, we can experience more of these beautiful moments. This book is designed to support you in your journey to collect and create more pearls of your own.

So let's get started.

Gander Reroute 9/11
By Diane and Nick Marson

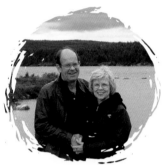

Diane:

Iwas flying from London to my hometown of Houston, having just visited my son who was stationed in England. Three hours into the flight, the pilot came over the intercom and announced that due to an emergency in the United States, we would be rerouted to Canada. I thought there was something wrong with the plane. But when we landed in Gander, a tiny town in Newfoundland on Canada's Northeast coast, we learned that multiple sites in the United States had been attacked, and that planes had been used as weapons. It was September 11, 2001.

I didn't have a cell phone, which didn't much matter, as other passengers' phones weren't working anyway. We watched as other planes circled overhead and began to gather on the tarmac. In total, thirty-eight diverted planes wound up on the runway—seven thousand passengers in all—where we all stayed for the next thirty hours. We were, after all, potential security risks; who knew if there were more terrorists on one of those planes? In those early hours, it was impossible to know just where the threat was coming from, or what other attacks were still on their way.

For an entire day and then some, we sat helplessly in our seats. We had no way of reaching anyone. Flight attendants showed us movies, and slowly information trickled in from the

few people on board who had working phones—there had
been multiple attacks and many casualties. That was really
all we knew. It was a harrowing experience. We had no way
to contact our loved ones, to learn if they were okay or to tell
them where we were. My son travels a great deal for business,
and not being able to reach him was the worst part. We were
scared, exhausted and dazed. The situation was so incredibly
surreal.

When we were finally able to get off the planes (with only
our carry-ons), we all needed to be checked. The process
took hours. The Red Cross and Salvation Army had to verify
our identities, give everyone their necessary medications and
guide us to our temporary shelters. We made our way into the
terminal for food, and then school buses transported us to our
destinations. It was obvious that the whole of Newfoundland
hadn't slept at all that night. From filling prescriptions, to
preparing food and bedding, they had it all covered.

Gander isn't a particularly wealthy town. It's also not very
large and certainly not large enough to accommodate seven
thousand stranded travelers. Its population is only around
eleven thousand. Yet none of the people seemed to mind that
we had descended upon their town, nearly doubling it in size
without notice. On the contrary, the people of Gander seemed
pleased to have us and eager to do whatever they could to
help make our stay comfortable. They took all of us in, making
us homemade food, putting us up in community buildings
and some even took us into their own homes. We were all so
scared, and I imagine they were too, seeing images of burning
buildings looped on the news. I think they felt sympathy for
Americans and were glad to have the chance to express it.

I wound up staying at the Society of United Fishermen
(S.U.F.), in a small town called Gambo, some 20 miles from
Gander, and that was where I met Nick.

We struck up a conversation while waiting in line for
blankets. He seemed friendly and sweet. There were only

about seventy or eighty of us in the lodge—most people stayed in Gander proper. Initially, I had been taken to the Salvation Army, but it turned out they were already full. I had been delayed trying to fill medication that had been in my suitcase. There were only five or six of us from the Houston flight in the lodge—the odds were very low that we would both find ourselves there, not to mention in Canada at all! Had we been able to take our checked luggage, we would probably not have met.

Having struck up a conversation in the morning, Nick and I ended up talking the rest of the evening and wound up in cots next to each other that first night. In the morning we went for a walk. It was a beautiful day, and we needed time away from the constant news. By now, I had reached my son and I was feeling a lot better. I wanted to stay in the park all afternoon so I bought us both Diet Coke and trail mix. I figured then Nick would have to stay and talk some more. Already I felt an attraction toward him, and I hoped he felt the same.

The next day one of the local school teachers generously took us to see Dover Fault—a well known geological site which marks the area where North American and European continents collided 150 million years ago.

Nick was taking pictures of the scenery, so I stepped out of his way.

"No," he said, "get back in the shot."

I did, and he took a photo of me. I realized at that point the feeling of attraction was mutual.

Finally, commercial airlines were allowed to fly again, and one by one, our planes were cleared to leave. Five days had passed since we landed in Newfoundland. As we began to head toward the school bus that would take us to the airport, I began to cry. It figures I'd meet a great guy here, this way and never see him again, I thought.

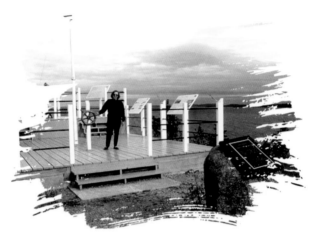

Nick put his arm around me and went to kiss me on the forehead. I kissed him on the lips instead. Time was running out, and I needed to show my intentions. I felt like a teenager with a bundle of mixed up emotions instead of a grandmother who had just celebrated her 60th birthday.

When we arrived at the airport, there was a rainbow. Was Nick the pot of gold at the end of it—the extraordinary gift I took from this whole strange and harrowing experience? Of course, I'm so grateful that we met. But I like to think that the real pot of gold was this amazing group of people: this town full of kind strangers who had no obligation to help us, and yet did, again and again, welcoming us into their homes and their hearts. They shut down their schools so people could sleep in them. The town bus drivers suspended their strike so they could transport us wherever we needed to go. Pharmacists arrived at the temporary shelters, offering their services and medications without any expectation of payment. One woman, risking her own life, searched all the planes and found nineteen animals including cats, dogs and two rare Bonobo chimpanzees. She put her life on hold for five days and cared for all of them!

Nick and I sat together on the flight to Houston. He stayed for a week, and we met up in the evenings. Then he had to return to England.

He visited again in October to check on a work project—or so he said. I believed that I was the project! As it turned out, I was right.

In November, Nick proposed over the phone.

He came back to Houston again in December and moved there permanently in May 2002. We were married on September 7, 2002, and we returned to Newfoundland for our honeymoon. We had booked a room in the Gander Hotel. And once again, everyone there was so incredibly kind—so welcoming, so glad to have us. They hadn't just been good to us because of the extenuating circumstances; they were wonderful to us because that was just how they are.

We celebrated with the families who had taken care of us, who had seen to our needs in a strange and scary time, and who had, whether they meant to or not, given us a beautiful—and safe, and comforting—place to fall in love.

Nick:

In 2001, I was working in the oil industry and had recently changed my job. My new company was doing some experimental drilling in Texas. Originally, I was set to fly out on September 10, but the necessary software was malfunctioning, so I stayed behind to help fix it and booked myself on a flight the next morning.

Diane was in the front of the plane, and I was in the rear, so we didn't meet until after we had deplaned on September 12. We were transported separately to the S.U.F. in Gambo, a nearby town. Schools, churches and public buildings had been converted into shelters for all of the stranded passengers. We met that evening while we were both in line to get a blanket. Diane cracked a little joke—something about mothballs or camphor or something. I joked back. I remember thinking, *"Well, she doesn't look too bad at all."* We were all very crammed in—it was a small building—and she and I slept beside each other that night. I had a good feeling about her, and of course being there alone and feeling so disoriented and isolated, it was comforting to have someone to talk to. Here we were, out of our element, and that's where I found this amazing woman.

There was a very odd feeling in the air. Despite all the generosity and sacrifice—a kind of compassion and selflessness I had never really seen before and haven't seen since—being stranded in Gander was intensely lonely. We had received news in pieces—we knew planes had been flown into buildings; we knew that people had died—when you hear news like that, all you want is to be with your family and never let go of them. You, at the very least, want to touch base to make certain that everyone you know and love is okay and to make sure they know that you, too, are okay. At first, there weren't enough phones to go around since everyone was so anxious to use one. But the good people of Gander called in workers to install more phones. They even turned the local school library into an 'Internet Café,' enabling everyone to make contact with their loved ones.

Even once we had made contact, we still felt such fear and uncertainty. When something that awful happens, you almost can't believe it. I was safe, but I still felt so sad and vulnerable whenever I thought about all the people who were injured and all those who had died. You didn't know if there were further attacks coming, or what else might happen in these days. And yet we were set down in this wonderful, peaceful place, where they were looking after us, and here was this woman who seemed so lovely.

The next morning, we all had breakfast together in the lodge. Diane looked beautiful in the midst of all that strangeness. Everyone was so incredibly welcoming and accommodating. It was overwhelming. One of the stranded passengers asked for green tea, which the lodge didn't have, so someone from the area sent her husband home to get it. It seems like such a small thing, but one I'll never forget. With all of the food, bedding, medication, phones, computers that needed to be gathered, it was clear that these wonderful people hadn't slept a wink since we all arrived.

On the first night there, the people of Gander threw a little party, called 'Screeching,' to cheer us up. We were all made honorary Newfoundlanders. The way one became an honorary Newfoundlander was to kiss a dead codfish, and you had to sing a song about where you were from. Diane sang, "Yellow Rose of Texas," and I sang, "I Am a Londoner." The master of ceremonies saw us together and assumed we were married. We said we weren't, and he asked if we wanted him to marry us. "Why not?" Diane said. I knew she was joking, but I also knew there was something there and thought that maybe this could work.

Out of the kindness of their hearts, they took us on trips during the day to help ease the stress.

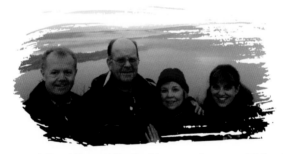

Lee MacDougal (l) and Sharon Wheatley (r), actors who portray Nick and Diane (center) in the Tony-winning Broadway Musical, *Come From Away*.

Soon, flights began to leave, but I really didn't want to go. We were in this heavenly place, and everyone had been so kind to us—but what I really wanted was to be with Diane. I remember thinking that I had no idea if I would ever get to see her again.

Luckily for me, she gave me her business card. Together with the picture that I had of her at Dover Fault, these were the most important things that I had as we were headed to the plane. We flew back to Houston together, and I stayed as long as I could before I had to return home. Back in England, I would take her card out and look at it. Checking the card ensured that I hadn't lost it and more importantly confirmed that this event really happened and I hadn't simply just dreamt it. I came back to Texas twice more to see her and knew very quickly that we wanted to remain together. When I asked her to marry me over the phone in November, she said "Yes." We both agreed there was only one place we could go on our honeymoon. Newfoundland.

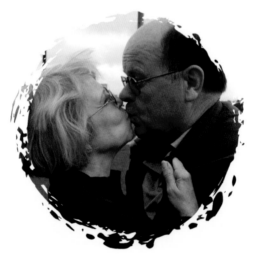

We planned to host a party to say 'A BIG THANK YOU' to all of our 'Newfie' family and friends. But no, these wonderful people did it again. When we arrived at our large wedding celebration at the S.U.F. in Gambo, we learned that we'd received all sorts of donations from local businesses. The local mayor, Lloyd Noseworthy, wrote and played a song about us, which our friend Amanda sang at the evening's festivities. They even had a wedding cake, gifts and a champagne toast.

It wasn't until later that we found out that only the head table had champagne; to save money, the rest of the tables had sparkling cider. We had so many presents that Diane had difficulty fitting them all into our luggage.

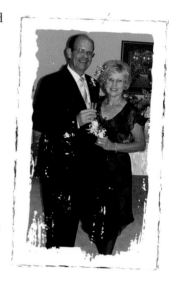

Diane and I both suffered from survivor's guilt, and for the longest time, we were not comfortable sharing our story with anyone outside of close family and friends. It felt strange that we had found so much happiness in the wake of such disaster and misery suffered by so many around the world. In this challenging time, an entire island of people came together to help whomever they could. And if they hadn't, I would never have found the love of my life.

In 2009, we were approached by NBC to be part of the Tom Brokaw "Operation Yellow Ribbon" documentary that was to be shown during the 2010 Winter Olympics in Canada. The show saluted the generosity and kindness of the Newfoundlanders. Diane and I are the "Autumn Romance." This program was seen by an Austrian film company who decided to take us back to Gander for the 10th anniversary, September 11, 2011. It was then that we met the Canadian husband and wife playwright team of David Hein and Irene Sankoff. They told us they were writing a musical about 9/11. Yes, really. This musical, *Come from Away*, is now a Tony Awards® winner on Broadway.

Diane and I have seen the show 58 times in six different cities and two different countries. We just keep going back. Every time we see the show, I believe that it strengthens our bond by taking us back to those five days in Newfoundland.

We love meeting the audience afterward—it's wonderful to see the effect that the show has had on them. I believe that it helps people heal from the damaging effects of 9/11. When we talk to them they tell us two things: where they were on 9/11, and how they met their partner. Every couple has their own special story—maybe a look, a cup of coffee, first dance, sitting together on a bus, first movie and their first kiss. My favorite story is the six-foot seven-inch basketball player with a five-foot wife. On their first date, this hunk of a guy was so frightened that he took his buddy along with him for support.

Diane and I have our own special story; sadly it happened when the world was in such turmoil. And now our story is included in this Broadway hit, quite unbelievable that this should happen to two ordinary people who found themselves in very extraordinary circumstances.

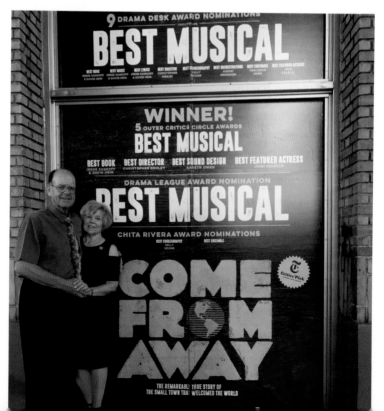

The Unlikely Savior
By Asheritah Ciuciu

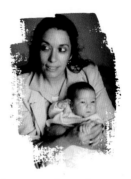

T he young woman swallowed hard as she tapped on the door.

"Come in," a voice said.

She wobbled into the office, trying to balance her pregnant belly as her knees knocked together. She saw a woman frowning at her across a desk.

"What do you want now?" the woman said.

"Can I talk to you privately?" the young woman asked, her voice trembling. The woman who had filed her deportation paperwork gave her a slight nod. Taking a deep breath and sending a quick prayer heavenward, the 21-year-old poured out her heart. This was her last chance to save her life and that of her unborn baby.

That young woman was my mother and that unborn baby was me.

In broken French mixed with English, my mother shared her story. Back home, in Romania, she had married a young, handsome pastor, and together they had served in a church. During their time there, there had been dramatic growth in the church's attendees, especially among the younger generation. The city's secret police took notice and began interrogating her husband, pressuring him to divulge the names of new converts, active church members, and Bible smugglers. When he refused, the police threatened him, and he soon faced death threats. She and her husband had been forced into hiding, planning to escape from the country with their two-year-old son. But only she had been granted a traveler's visa. So she boarded a plane to visit her uncle in Israel, and after failing to secure political asylum there, boarded another plane to the nearest country that offered asylum: Greece.

Tears trickled down my mother's face as she showed pictures of her loved ones trapped behind the Iron Curtain. "Please," she asked. "Please help us. If you send me back now, they'll throw me in prison and I'll never see them or my baby again."

The external transit officer watched my mother rub her pregnant belly, dabbing her eyes with a tissue. She had stayed two hours past her shift at the airport's immigration department as it was, and almost certainly longed to kick off her high heels and relax at home. But something about this young woman's demeanor softened her composure, and she did the unthinkable: halted the deportation process and threw all her energy into saving this young woman's life.

She picked up the phone and, in rapid Greek, spoke first to the Immigration Director at the airport, then to the International Migration Catholic Institute Director, then to an old pal at the Athens police, and finally to a member of the United Nations. Within an hour she had contacted the four people who could adjust my mother's status to political refugee, and, in the weeks that followed, she placed her in a crisis pregnancy center, then later intervened to help her keep me despite the center's policies that demanded babies be given up for adoption.

That transit officer became my honorary godmother and secured an apartment right above her own for my mother and me—this pair that had made their way into her heart. She also arranged for cleaning jobs so that my mother could buy food and basic necessities, and she continued pressuring the UN to assist my father and brother as well. Seven months after that fortunate encounter in her small airport office, she witnessed our family's reunion, and eleven months later, bid us goodbye as we continued our journey to the United States.

This woman's act of kindness that day saved both my life and that of my family, and her influence continues to bless us to this day, across so many years and continents and oceans.

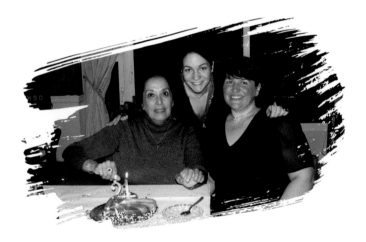

"Kindness, I've discovered, is everything in life."

—Isaac Bashevis Singer

A Generous Heart
By Allan Varah

I couldn't sleep—rare for me, but then again, so was this pain. Maybe TV will help, I thought, as I dragged myself towards the living room. Breath short, chest tight, mind blurred—what the hell was going on? It was my third day of discomfort and only getting worse. As if my whole upper body was rebelling, even breathing was now a real challenge. Climbing stairs or walking the crowded city streets earlier left me winded. What a mess!

I looked at the clock's red glow: 2:00 a.m. 2:01…2:02… Listening to my shallow breath, my mind unfocused, I wondered: Am I going to die? Anti-alarmist to the bone, I felt a very real, unfamiliar worry build within me.

New to New York City, having only left happy-go-lucky Canadian medicine a few months earlier, I was both uninsured and afraid. Young, poor and otherwise uptight about money— especially the sort I didn't have—I prayed this would all pass. Pass, damn it!! Pass!!

But as the minutes ticked by, the pain worsened, and I grew more scared. "Breaking News" showed bloodstained car seats on TV. Princess Diana had just been in an accident. Was it a sign? Regardless, I had had enough. Day and night, ambulances roared down Lexington or across 77th, and now for the first time I followed the siren's call, grabbed my shoes and made my way to the Lenox Hill Hospital. Weak and disoriented, feet dragging cinder blocks, I lumbered inside.

I filled out an intake form, sat in the Emergency Room waiting room panting shallow breaths, trying to stay calm, until I was called in.

Five minutes into it I'm covered in stickies, hooked-up to a heart monitor. Five minutes more, and in came the questions.

"How much cocaine do you do?" the woman asked.

"Huh? What?? None," I said.

"You work on Wall Street?" She pressed.

"Yes, but what does that mean?"

"Well, from what I'm seeing, you've got a nasty little heart condition on your hands. Can't say we see many twenty-one-year-olds looking like you do. I'll get the cardiologist to explain."

My fears receded—they knew what was going on, definitely a comfort, even if what was going on was a "nasty little heart condition."

In walks a young, well-groomed doctor. "You have a textbook case of Pericarditis," he tells me. "It's an inflammation of the lining surrounding the heart. Mimics a heart attack. Can be life threatening, but rarely is. Just the same, it's miserable and absolutely needs medical attention. I'm going to keep you overnight—be sure the meds get this under control."

I stayed quiet.

"Nurse shared that you're on day three feeling like this. Tough guy, huh? What took you so long to come in?"

"I don't have health insurance."

"And you were going to risk death to save some money?"

Back to being quiet.

"Well, tell you what, I was young and new to New York once, too. I can't prevent the hospital from billing you for the bed, but I won't put in for my time. Good news is: I'm the expensive part."

I smiled and thanked him. Not the way I should have—not in the "holy cow, you're easily the greatest doctor ever" way. Or the "wow!! you're willing to break protocol for the sake of my financial vulnerability!!!" way. Even worse, he came back for several check-ups and reassured me all was going to be okay, and each time I said very little. Full of gratitude, but shy, uncommunicative me stayed quiet.

If that wasn't bad enough, I never went back after recovering. I lived across the street and didn't so much as drop in to say: "Look at me Doc! I'm better, and you're my hero!" Something about being awkward and otherwise in my own world, I guess.

So, as I write this, however long the odds that it'll reach the intended audience, here's what I'd like to say to that incredibly kind doctor who guided me back to health and stuck his neck out along the way: you saw a scared, poor kid, shaking in his boots, and you did everything possible to help. To put it simply: thank you, thank you, THANK YOU! Not just for the financial part of things, but for the reassurance, compassion, and the time you took to help me see that, pain and fear aside, everything was going to be okay. It was beautiful and kind, and for that, I will be forever grateful.

> "The life so short, the craft so long to learn."
>
> —*Hippocrates*

Two Tears
By Christopher Malec

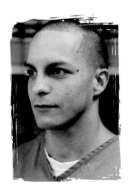

The memory is a blur to me, and most of what I do remember feels like something I watched through someone else's eyes. I recall being loaded onto the long, steel Bluebird bus in a line of slumped shadows with sunken heads. It was still dark outside—chillier than usual for Florida, it seemed to me—and the metal shackles around my ankles made me all the more aware of the cold.

The long ride through early-morning traffic to the courthouse would be like many I had taken in the twenty-one months leading up to this day. I was surrounded by chatter from a group of equally apprehensive souls, each wondering whether or not it would be the day freedom rang. There were no windows, save for the driver's. The hard plastic seats seemed to grow harder with every bump in the road.

When I reached the holding cell beneath the courtrooms, time seemed to go more slowly. I knew what was coming. I spent hours curled up on a bench, my head resting against the pale yellow wall where a hundred names had been carved— people who'd sat there just like me.

Once I made it into the courtroom, things moved quickly: impeccable suits disputing my fate, a judge banging the familiar wooden hammer, saying what I knew he would: "Life."

I had lost at trial a month before and had known ever since that this would be my sentence. I had even called home and told everyone to prepare for it. I didn't shed any tears. In fact, I smirked in disbelief that the system claimed to serve justice: Justice had not prevailed in this room.

And then I felt a gentle hand on my shoulder and looked up to meet the eyes of a bailiff who had seen me in countless courtrooms since I was a teenager. There were tears streaming down her cheeks. I had no family in the courtroom, no friends, and here she was, shedding tears for me as if I were her own. My own eyes watered. I sucked it up, determined to be strong. Not just for me, but for her and anyone else like her. She made me decide that very moment to never give up the fight, no matter how long or exhausting.

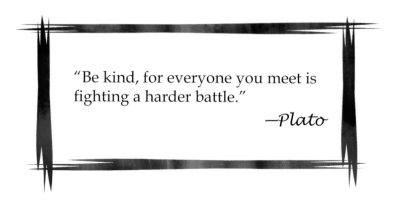

"Be kind, for everyone you meet is fighting a harder battle."

—Plato

My Lucky Day
By Jane Goldberg

It was a frigid Saturday morning and a friend of mine invited me to the Tribeca Synagogue. I participated in the *Kiddush* (a blessing recited over a cup of wine or bread) following the prayer service. This particular synagogue is on White Street and it is white white white! It sticks out like a piece of modern art, set way back from the street, and is surrounded by old, cast-iron buildings. There are a few sculptures off to the side, like castaways, perfect for locking up my bike which I rode there.

As a tap dancer and performance historian, I have commuted everywhere I needed to go in New York City by bicycle since 1974. I get places fast and stay in shape!

After the *Kiddush*, I went back outside into the freezing cold, unlocked my bike and headed south toward the Statue of Liberty to the A train at Church and Chambers Streets, only a few blocks away. When I got to a pole near the subway where I was going to lock my bike, I discovered, after furiously rummaging through my purse, I couldn't find my keys! NOT AGAIN! Was this *déjà vu* or, worse, a recurring nightmare? My first instinct was denial. That would have been the third time I'd lost a set of keys that week!

After a few minutes of shivering in the cold, searching through my purse again and emptying all its contents on the sidewalk, I rode back to the Tribeca Synagogue taking the exact same route I took to the subway. Surely, I had dropped them by the sculpture where I parked my bike. But no, *nada*, no keys anywhere. We New Yorkers tend to overlook the homeless people begging on the streets, panhandling, and often, even in the winter, asleep under a lot of blankets, but they are always there. We often choose not to see them, a fixture, like some huge blight to the city. There are city shelters. Why sit outside in the freezing cold, I often wonder? But the weather doesn't stop them from begging or waiting for a hand out, even on a frigid winter day.

So, when I passed an old, disheveled-looking man sitting on a metal chair, with a little plastic cup in front of him with hardly any change in it, I didn't think much about it. That is, not until he screamed out to no one in particular, "Life isn't worth living!!!! What's the use?"

Those words resonated with me from head to toe, especially given my own immediate despair. I didn't look back, but when I got to the corner of the next block, I stopped and began to look for some loose change.

Searching through my wallet, I found three ten-dollar bills, but not one penny, nickel, dime, or quarter! I must have stood on that corner for over five minutes deliberating what to do. A ten-dollar bill was a lot for me to give to a panhandling stranger.

I had given up the key search having already covered my trail numerous times. I was going to have to take my bike onto the subway. But before I did, I walked back toward the old man, recalling his outcry of despair and handed him one of my ten-dollar bills, and I said off the cuff, "This is your lucky day and my unlucky day."

He immediately stood up and said, "I don't want this to be your unlucky day." I waved him off as I started to leave, saying, "It's not your fault…I lost my keys,…again."

The old man turned around, and from a standpipe* behind him, picked up my keys and showed them to me, asking, "Are these yours?" Indeed, they were! Shocked at the sight

*Standpipes, vertical pipes connected to a water supply, are still standing all over the New York City manufacturing districts and other parts of the city. They were once used to help put out fires, replaced by fire hydrants. Now they're just there, standing, as symbols of a bygone era in New York City.

of my keys, I couldn't believe my eyes! It was like the Red Sea had parted. I had just come from the Synagogue and this unexpected miracle had happened. How could this be? There I was hesitating, hemming and hawing, about my ten-dollar bills and no change. Not impulsively, I made the decision to give him the money and in return he gave me a priceless gift.

An additional gift on his part was pointing out to me a gigantic mural on a dirty white wall across the street. The mural was in plain view, so very big, unobscured by scaffolding and the other construction equipment occupying so much of New York City these days. I had completely missed seeing it as I was so caught up in my own head, which was swirling with a combination of worry and self-criticism. The man told me those multicultural faces of children and adults were portraits of the first people to land on Ellis Island, the gateway for many millions of immigrants coming to the United States. He shared with me that he had always been interested in history.

I was so grateful that he had found my keys, I asked him if he needed anything. Then I glanced down and saw the dilapidated shoes he was wearing. He told me what he really needed was a warm coat. I vowed to find him one…and I did.

There are multiple lessons I drew from this cosmic coincidence: I should be less self-critical for losing my keys… and that life can be easier and happier by giving and accepting kind gestures from strangers. I think this should be true for all of us.

> "The best way to find yourself is to lose yourself in the service of others."
> —Mahatma Gandhi

Doctor's Orders
By Rosalinda Chavez

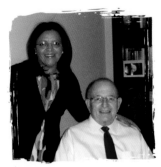

I was born in Honduras and grew up in a very poor community. My mother, a strong woman with an equally strong faith in God, taught me that every person, no matter how rich or poor, is equal. Nobody is any better than anyone else, she would tell me. I came to America and worked for many wealthy families, and I struggled to believe what my mother taught me. It seemed that in America, the rich were valued more than the poor. But when my former boss introduced me to her friend, who introduced me to her dad, I knew my mother was right.

Dr. Kline is one of the kindest men I have ever met. He showed me that being kind meant treating every person the way I wanted to be treated. Dr. Kline treated his patients, his residents, his friends, his family and even strangers he met in an equally kind fashion. God blessed me when he brought me to Dr. Kline and allowed me to serve as his wife's caretaker, then as his, from his initial diagnosis of Parkinson's to his passing. He was like a father to me. He loved and guided me like one of his own daughters.

I realized how kind Dr. Kline was when I watched him care for his wife while she was ill and dying. At the time, I was working as an aide for Mrs. Kline in Miami. She was very sick with a lung disease. When they decided that they wanted to go back home to Pittsburgh, I went with them. We rented a van so that Mrs. Kline would be comfortable and Dr. Kline stayed by his wife's side. She was in bed the whole trip. He taught me how important it was to pay attention to details. I watched him carefully when he massaged her hands and feet, gave her medications and monitored her oxygen. He stayed by her side and cared for her until she passed away.

Dr. Kline encouraged me to become a certified nurse. Because of his belief in my abilities, I started my nursing studies and my whole world opened up. He helped me understand the class material and spent hours teaching me. Every morning, we would eat together and talk about my life, my family back home in Honduras and my dreams. He was concerned about my family in Honduras, and he encouraged me to bring them to America. Every month he would give me extra money for my mother. And he would double-check to make sure I had sent it. Since I could not bring my whole family here, he sent me to Honduras so I could see my mother and family. During our long breakfast talks, he helped me learn English. We played Scrabble almost every day. He was so patient. Although he did not like to lose, I know he was proud of me on the rare occasions when I beat him!

I asked my husband whether we should move permanently to Pittsburgh. I wasn't sure if it was the right choice for us. I asked Dr. Kline what he thought. He encouraged me to stay in Pennsylvania. He pointed out that I did not have family in Miami, and that I was part of his family now. He asked if I needed money for a down payment. He paid for my husband to come to Pittsburgh to see the house I had picked out. He loved it, and we resettled in Pittsburgh. I was able to buy my first home in America.

There are so many other kind things that Dr. Kline did for me and my family. My son, Raul, is getting his Master's degree in renewable energy; he graduates in a month. Dr. Kline paid the initial installment to the university. He always expressed his gratitude for the work I did for him and his wife. He made me believe in myself and all that I could accomplish.

I think the kindest thing he did was to teach me so many of life's most important lessons. He taught me how to be a better parent. He taught me that the time and attention I give my children will always result in great joy for me and my husband.

The day before Dr. Kline died, I was shaving his face. He was in and out of consciousness. I told him, "I am here with you," and asked him to show a sign that he could hear me.

He took my hand and held it close.

That is what it was like for me to know him: I always felt that he was holding my hand, lovingly guiding me to be my best self.

"Kindness is the only service that will stand the storm of life and not wash out. It will wear well and will be remembered long after the prism of politeness or the complexion of courtesy has faded away."

—Abraham Lincoln

Three Strangers
By Sharni Montgomery

I was returning from a stroll, after reading the morning paper down in Coogee Beach, in Sydney, Australia. I noticed a man on the brink of what looked like a heart attack. He was clenching his chest, wobbling over the footpath and heading to a tree which he gripped onto.

I felt my insides freeze up. I looked around the main street of Coogee to find that I was the only person in the immediate vicinity.

Panic. This one was mine. I rushed over to the man.

"Are you OK?" I asked. Clearly, he wasn't.

"Is it your chest?" I asked.

He grabbed onto me, his whole body was shaking, he was heavy.

I looked around for help.

"Shall I call an ambulance?" I said.

"No, no," he said.

"Are you sure?" I was freaked, grabbed my phone with one hand, "I'm calling an ambulance."

"No, not an ambulance, just help me home," he said shaking, leaning on me, pale as a ghost, stinking.

Somebody else was rushing to my aide. An American tourist with a busted nose. He asked the stricken man some more questions. The man assured us he would be okay if we could just help him home. I held onto one side of the man, and the American tourist held the other side.

"Where do you live?" I asked.

"Just up here," he stammered in an Irish accent.

So the Aussie, the Irishman and the American all walked slowly towards the house he referred to.

Luckily it was not far. As he went for his keys his hands shook so much he could not retrieve them.

"You'll have to get them out of my pocket," he said to the American tourist.

As the door flung open, a strong smell of what could only be described as stale urine greeted us. I was gagging on the inside. We took him over to a chair.

His house was filthy. As he sat down, the American tourist and I looked at each other.

"Should we call an ambulance?" I asked him.

"Look, mate," he said, "You need to see a doctor."

"No, no doctor," he said. "Could you just get me a beer from the fridge love?" he said to me.

All of a sudden, it became clear what the trouble was.

I looked around his house for signs of family members.

"Does anyone else live here?" I asked.

"Just me."

I went to the fridge containing one long neck of VB (Victoria Bitter, a popular Australian beer) and not much else. I took it to the man whose shaking hands received it as though I was giving him water in the desert. He drank it full pelt.

Just like that his shaking subsided and color returned to his cheeks.

"Have a seat," he said to the American tourist and me.

We looked at each other uncomfortably and sat down. Too concerned to leave the stranger and unsure what to do next.

"What happened to your nose?" I asked the American tourist.

"Got belted at the Palace last night," he said.

The Irishman laughed.

"Is it broken?" the Irishman asked.

"Yep."

"Big night out then?" I asked

"Huge, can't even remember it," the American tourist said.

"I'm a bit hungover myself," I confessed.

At that moment it was as though the Universe was issuing me a tutorial on the evils of drinking.

That day, as three strangers sat in a smelly house together, I was face to face with the not-so-fun side of it. We all sat there together, hearing stories from each other's lives, awkwardly, for over an hour. When we were as sure as we could be that the Irishman was OK, we went our separate ways.

Every time I passed that house, I wondered if the Irishman was OK.

I still wonder.

It was one of those experiences so random I am sure it happened for a reason.

Three strangers in Coogee united in varying states of alcohol-inflicted pain, never to meet again, but never to forget their meeting.

"Kindness is the golden chain by which society is bound together."

—Johann Wolfgang von Goethe

Yes, Please
By Erika Irene Goodrich

The day I met Kiki, I had been forced to decline an invitation to a writing retreat in Barcelona—one that would have allowed me ten days of one-on-one mentoring with a well-known poet in one of the most beautiful cities in the world. It had been the opportunity of a lifetime. But my husband was interviewing for a job that would have had us moving the week of the retreat, which rendered the retreat impossible. (In the end, he didn't get the job—which would only double my disappointment.)

I set out that afternoon to run errands, hoping to distract myself. One task on my list was food shopping. As I drove to my local Publix Market, Florida's unrelenting sunshine glinted on the hood of my Jeep. All I could think about was what I was losing out on. At the market, I walked the aisles, daydreaming about the Mediterranean and the architecture of Gaudí.

When I finished, I placed the items one by one onto the conveyor belt: lettuce. Beep. Two cucumbers. Beep. Beep. Turkey breast. Beep.

"I love your shoes! Are they comfortable?" the wide-eyed Publix bagger asked. Her nametag read Kiki.

"Thanks," I said. "Yes, they are." I looked at my five-toe sneakers, willing the conversation to end soon.

"Your feet look so cute in them! Not everybody can wear those. Lots of people have ugly feet. Where did you get them?"

"Ebay, I think." My tone was terse. "Maybe 6pm.com—I don't know."

"Do you need special socks? Do you run in them? Are they better for walking? Do your feet get hot, compared to regular sneakers?"

"Yeah, you need toe-socks. They cost about twelve dollars a pair." I prayed she would stop talking.

"Wow!" she said. "That's crazy expensive. How much do the sneakers cost?"

Oh my, what else is this girl going to ask? I gritted my teeth, aware that I might be wearing my emotions on my sleeve. I didn't want to offend her—I just wanted to mourn in peace. But Kiki just went on and on, oblivious.

Then she handed me the receipt. I was ready to answer when she asked if I needed help out to my car: no thanks. Except Kiki never asked. She already had her hands on the cart's handle, and before I could speak, she

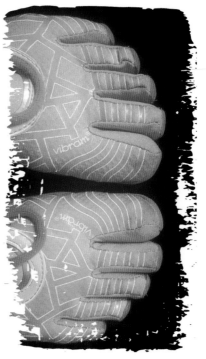

was rolling toward the door. For a split second, I thought of hijacking the cart and running toward my car.

But instead, with great reluctance, I walked with her toward my Jeep. I pointed left as Kiki steered. Fumbling through my purse, I grabbed my keys.

"Whew! It is hot out here," Kiki said.

I wondered why this girl had been so insistent about walking me to my car in ninety-degree heat.

I still don't know why, but from nowhere came a sudden thought—I remembered my yoga instructor's wise words. The emphasis she placed on the importance of being present, of tapping into the breath and being fully engaged in the moment, allowing love and beauty to shine through.

My day had been consumed by disappointment, and my first impulse in the face of that disappointment was to wallow in my misery, not interested in acknowledging anyone else. But when I tuned in to my breath, my focus shifted away from myself, and I started to wonder about Kiki's insistence. Was she bored? Lonely? Surely this wasn't all just about my sneakers. In that moment, when I became fully present, my jaw unclenched. I started to open like a flower leaning toward the warmth of the sun. Something inside me had shifted.

Kiki and I continued to chat about everything and nothing— skincare and makeup, sneakers, Florida and it's incredible heat. We talked beside my Jeep for what felt like hours. By then, I was so engaged in our conversation that time stood still, and we went on giggling like two old friends reunited after many years apart.

Finally, Kiki had to get back. She thanked me for the conversation. I continued to think about her on the drive home. I was so grateful that she didn't give me the chance to say "No thanks," at a time when I would have benefited from saying "Yes, please." It was her small act of kindness—a simple acknowledgment of me, an openness that opened me, in turn—that altered the direction of my day.

> "Kindness is like snow — it beautifies everything it covers."
>
> —Kahlil Gibran

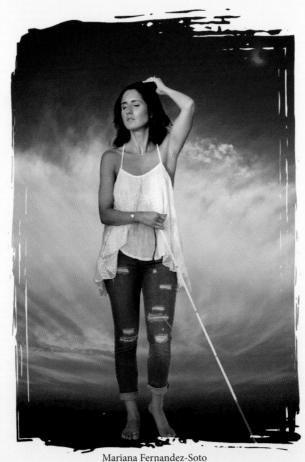

Mariana Fernandez-Soto
Marriage and Family Therapist
Photographed by Irina Lawton for the Bold Beauty Project, Miami, 2016

Beethoven

Beethoven wrote the song "Moonlight Sonata" because he wanted to give something to a blind girl he had met. She could not see the beauty around her. The white clouds, trees and colorful flowers were among the many beautiful sights she was not able to view. Beethoven sat down and put his genius to work, so she could hear the wondrous beauty in his composition.

Spreading Joy
By Georgia A. Hubley

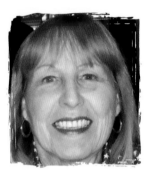

I was a multitasking mom with a family, home and a job I loved. Life was grand. Then the unthinkable happened, and I had to have emergency surgery. To my dismay, I was benched—sidelined for six weeks. My doctor's orders were as follows: no driving, no strenuous activity, no heavy lifting and lots of bed rest.

On the first day of sick leave, I rested, read a book and felt sorry for myself. However, on the second day, the mail carrier filled my mailbox with sunshine. When I opened the mailbox, I was elated to find six envelopes in various sizes and colors, all decorated with stickers and addressed to me in cursive. My co-workers had sent get-well and thinking-of-you cards. Their words of encouragement lifted my spirits.

For the next two weeks, my colleagues continued to send me these special cards, which arrived roughly every two days. Needless to say, the mail carrier's visit was my favorite time of day.

Then, three weeks into my convalescence, the cards stopped coming. My heart sank each time I opened the mailbox and only found bills, magazines or junk. Of course, it couldn't have lasted forever, I told myself. People get on with their lives.

But then the following week, the doorbell rang. I was flabbergasted when the mail carrier handed me a stack of bundled mail and said, chuckling, "You hit the mail jackpot. There's not enough room in your mailbox!"

After I thanked him and closed the door, a wave of anticipation surged through me. As I sorted through the cards, I noticed the postmarks varied greatly. For some unknown reason, the cards had been delayed in the mailroom and then released all at once.

The remaining weeks passed quickly, and the doctor was pleased with my recovery, giving me permission to return to work. I attributed my speedy recovery to those quirky, humorous cards. They had made my recovery bearable, brightening each day. I vowed that if anyone I knew was ever sidelined due to illness or injury, I'd help them fend off boredom and loneliness with a deluge of cards, the funnier the better.

I've kept that promise. Over the years, I've sent hundreds of cards to family and friends who've needed a little dose of delight in their lives. Of course, emails, e-cards and greeting cards aren't a cure-all. Several years ago, when a dear friend was diagnosed with a terminal illness, I wasn't certain if I should send her cards. Would they only upset her? However, she never lost her delightful sense of humor. I'd sit by her bedside or talk to her on the phone as she howled over the latest crazy card she'd received from me.

"Keep them coming!" she said. "They bring me so much joy." It was gratifying to hear her laugh.

I admit my guilty pleasure is still snail mail. Yes, even in this high-tech, high-speed electronic age, nothing makes me happier than an overflowing mailbox. It's rewarding to know my greeting cards are appreciated by family and friends. I know how much I appreciated them. I'll always be grateful for the kindness bestowed upon me during my lengthy convalescence. It's made me absolutely certain that joy can heal one's body, mind and spirit.

Forever Striving
By Roy Castro

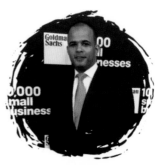

I was born and raised in the Bronx. Growing up in New York City, I fell onto hard times. My father was absent, and my mother was addicted to crack. I adopted the lifestyle of the streets. I was incarcerated for selling drugs and ended up doing a little over ten years in prison.

When I was inside, a man named Jose Ramos took an interest in me. He was the one who got me into education. He pushed me to get a GED. He didn't know me; I didn't know him. But he took a liking to me. He saw I was rough around the edges, and he sat me down and really guided me to start looking at life from the right perspective.

Jose got me a book, *The Seven Habits of Highly Effective People* by Stephen Covey. He taught me about stocks and bonds. He took it upon himself to educate me about the ways of the world and the things I needed to know to be successful. He made me feel differently about myself: Wow, I thought, I'm not stupid. I can learn. I like books. I like to read. I like being smart.

Most days, instead of hanging out with the other inmates, I was in my cell reading, bettering myself and preparing for my release. Jose and I lost contact—things happen in there, you wake up one morning and people are just gone, moved somewhere else without any warning. There's no rhyme or reason to it.

Upon my release, I tried to find a job. I went to interview after interview, but kept getting turned down—I was an eight-time convicted felon. After a few weeks, I even went and spoke to a friend about selling drugs again. I was so frustrated I didn't know what else to do. My friend's mother overheard me talking. She said, "Hey, listen, there's a program named STRIVE International and before you do anything silly, go give STRIVE a chance." She gave me the address, and I went and applied.

The woman at the front desk took my application and said, "Go sit down, class is about to start in a few minutes. You're going to be in orientation."

I thought about Jose—he was such a kind person, with a good spirit about him. Meeting him was the turning point in my life. He would have been so proud to see me there, at STRIVE, sitting in a class. STRIVE picked up where he left off. They taught me what it takes to find employment and to keep it. They taught me how to use a computer and how to exist in the world.

When I left STRIVE, I got a job cleaning freezers for an ice cream company. I worked my way up to be the manager. Then I started my own business—another ice cream company. Now we distribute all over the northeast.

I read constantly. Jose always said that the best way to learn is to teach, so every time I read a book, I find someone to teach what I learned. Sometimes it's my wife or my child. Other times, it is my employees or my business partner.

Jose taught me that you should always be kind. You should treat people the way you would like to be treated. It's about giving; it's about paying it forward. That's where I'm at in my life. Anybody I meet and I can give help to, I give it because so much was given to me. I've made it my mission to speak positivity to everyone, to be kind and to inspire.

Celebrating Kindness

Every day is the perfect day to be kind, but there are some you may not want to miss:

National Random Acts of Kindness Day: February 17 and World Kindness Day: November 13 each year.

National Random Acts of Kindness Day started in Denver, Colorado in 1995 and spread to New Zealand in 2004. This global celebration is easy to participate in. Simply perform one random act of kindness, and share it on social media, #RandomActsOfKindnessDay, or donate to Project Wilderness, and they will carry out your random act of kindness.

World Kindness Day is a global, twenty-four-hour celebration dedicated to paying it forward and focusing on the good. It was introduced in 1998 by the World Kindness Movement, a coalition of kindness NGO's (non-government organizations). It is observed in many countries, including the UK, Canada, Japan, Australia, Nigeria, United Arab Emirates, Singapore, Italy and India. It is a day that encourages individuals to overlook boundaries, race and religion. Events include The Big Hug, Handing out Kindness Cards, and a Global Flashmob, coordinated by Orly Wahba, kindness guru and founder of Life Vest Inside. The most recent flash mob, in 2016, was held in fifteen countries in thirty-three cities, and images were displayed in Time Square.

Mark your calendars now. These days will serve as positive reminders to bring more kindness into your life and to those around you.

Italian Ice and a Dollar
By Laquantis Morton

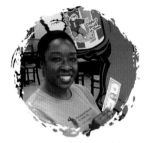

I was having lunch outdoors not too long ago when an older gentleman came up to me. He appeared to be homeless, and he asked me if I had any extra food. Unfortunately, I had just finished my meal and had started enjoying the Italian ice I'd ordered for dessert. I told him this, and he walked away, mumbling.

But then I had an idea—I decided to offer him my Italian ice. "Hey!" I said. "You can have my Italian ice."

The man turned and looked back, then returned to my table and said, "That isn't food." I said, "Well, this is all I have."

He said okay and took it and sat down with me. We began talking about our lives. He asked me where I was from and what I did; I asked how his day was going. We laughed. He pulled a dollar from his pocket and reached out to give it to me.

"No, no," I said, "you keep that."

"No, no," he said, "you take it."

We went back and forth a few times until finally, I said I would take it and give it to someone who needed it. He nodded and stood up, and I noticed it was time for me to catch my train. We said our goodbyes, and that was that.

But when I left, I kept thinking about that man and his act of dignity and respect. I had offered what little I had, and so had he.

I keep that dollar with me, to always remind myself to be open to whoever passes through my life—and to never question the way in which kindness is given in the world.

Giving in America

Americans have a long history of charitable giving and are becoming increasingly generous over time.

In 2016, CAF (Charities Aid Foundation) World Giving Index, surveyed approximately 1000 people in 140 countries. The U.S. ranked second in the world in charitable giving: 63% of the people surveyed said they had given money, 73% reported they had helped a stranger, and 46% percent said they had volunteered in the last month. Myanmar (formerly known as Burma) took first

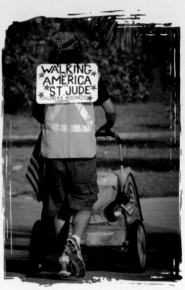

© Sandra Döhnert

place for the third year in a row: ninety-one percent of people said they donated money in the month prior and 63% said they had helped a stranger. Completing the top ten list were Australia, New Zealand, Sri Lanka, Canada, Indonesia, the UK, Ireland and the United Arab Emirates. The most common form of giving was helping a stranger. Iraq came in first in that category with 81% saying they had helped within the last month. For the first time since CAF began surveying in 2010, *over one-half of the people globally said they had helped a stranger within the last month.*

In June 2010, the Giving Pledge was formally announced by Bill Gates and Warren Buffett, and they began recruiting members. Its mission is to encourage the world's wealthiest individuals and families to dedicate the majority of their wealth to philanthropic causes. The pledge does not involve pooling any money or committing to any specific cause. By June 2016, 154 individuals and/or couples from 16 countries had pledged to give away $732 billion during their lifetime or in their wills.

Before you donate, you may want to learn more about the charities that interest you. Charity Navigator (charitynavigator. org), founded in 2001, has become the nation's largest and most-utilized evaluator of charities. It has developed a rating system and can provide you information about a charity's financial health, accountability and transparency. Charity Navigator has evaluated over 8,350 charities and provides users with a wide range of information including the tax benefits of donating, how to donate non-cash items and a guide to volunteering. GuideStar is another valuable source for information about nonprofits. They provide information and access to 1.8 million IRS-recognized tax-exempt organizations. JustGive is one of a growing number of websites, which for a minimal fee, will process donations for people wishing to give to charities online. The JustGive Guide has a nineteen-category collection of 1,000 recommended charities. It's best to do your homework so you can make not only kind, but also wise decisions.

> "I don't think you ever stop giving. I really don't. I think it's an ongoing process. And it's not just about being able to write a check. It's being able to touch somebody's life."
>
> —Oprah Winfrey

Many Kinds of Kindness
By Shirley Press

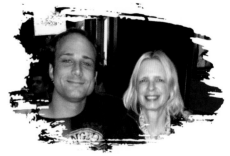

Kindness comes in many forms. These include giving money, giving of oneself, and doing good deeds, to name just a few. I've had the good fortune over my life of being on the giving and receiving end of many of these forms.

In 2001, while working as the head of a pediatric emergency room, I won the Florida Lottery. As a physician, I'd had the satisfaction of helping children and their parents for many years, and I viewed the lottery win as an opportunity to do even more.

About a year after the lottery, I reduced my work to part-time, and armed with the winnings, my husband and I began making changes. First, I made sure my family was taken care of. I asked my mother what she wanted most. Her reply: a new refrigerator. So I bought that for her, along with a new car. I gave my sister and first cousins money for college educations, and once we had set aside some money for other family needs, we found many worthy projects to support.

Over these past years, we've been very grateful for the opportunities we have had, but we've also learned, painfully, that there are so many issues that can't be solved with money alone.

My son, Gershon, has struggled with drug addiction since he was nineteen years old. He is now thirty-two. This is not only his struggle; it is our family's struggle, too. It has opened my eyes to this plight, which is all too common. It has also changed the way that I view drug addiction. I used to feel that it was the user's fault—it was just a matter of self-control. This is wrong in every sense. It is a disease, and blaming the sufferer is completely incorrect. My son's gritty world has been an eye-opener. I've met all kinds of people I would have never met in my life if not for him and this disease.

A few years ago, Gershon was arrested for possession of crack (the charges were later dropped). He was living in a halfway house after spending five and a half weeks in jail. For him, the halfway house provided relative freedom before he was to enter a rehabilitation facility. Gershon has a pattern of being self-destructive and often gives up on things at the last minute. On the day he was supposed to be transferred to rehab, I woke early to pick him up and drive him to the rehab van. Even though the van stop was only ten minutes away from the halfway house, I feared that he would never get onto it and miss an important opportunity for treatment. When I arrived, I was surprised and happy to see that Gershon was ready. We were carrying his bags to the car when he told me that he had to make another trip back to the room to pick up his radio.

I said, "No, just leave it," for fear that he would bolt.

My heart sank. I panicked. I was afraid of what was going to happen next.

He finished placing his stuff in the car and was about to return to his room when his roommate greeted him with the radio. Having no other choice, Gershon got into the car, and we sped away.

With tears in my eyes, I mouthed, "Thank you."

Whether he knew it or not, my son's roommate spared our family from possible disaster. Such a small gesture, such a small act of kindness, was a game-changer for my son and meant the absolute world to me. It reminded me that all acts have consequences, and sometimes the smallest acts of kindness have the greatest positive impact on those on the receiving end.

We're Kindness Powered

By Jennifer Bright Reich

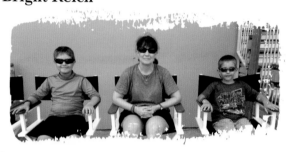

You might have seen the movie "Monsters, Inc.," where the company—in fact, the entire town—is powered by screams. My company, on the other hand, is entirely powered by the kindness of strangers.

In 2006, I was talking with a book-editor friend who had just landed a plum job with a huge New York publisher; it was her job to acquire books written in series. "So, Jennifer, if you ever have any book series ideas, let me know!" she said breezily. In that instant, a tiny thought that had been in the back of my mind for a few years raced to the surface! Yes, actually, I did have an idea. I had long been fascinated by tips that doctors who are also mothers used for their own families. I'd long thought their advice must be the best of the best. They're experts—squared, drawing from their experience as physicians and their wisdom as mothers.

I reached out to the kindest doctor I'd ever met, Dr. Rallie McAllister, who said she'd love to join me on the project. That Mother's Day, she shocked me by suggesting we start our own company and publish the books ourselves. We started to reach out to doctors, and we were surprised and grateful for their responses. These women—arguably some of the busiest women on the planet—graciously gave us their time, many of them again and again as our book list grew.

Since 2006, our company has grown to include more than 150 Mommy MD Guides! These doctors are from all over the country, and I've only met four of them in person. We've sold thousands of copies of the Mommy MD Guides books, which means these 150+ kind strangers have gone on to help thousands of other strangers. We are now published in multiple countries and I'm over-the-moon happy to think that our words and guidance will help moms a world away.

"Throw kindness around like confetti."

—Bob Goff

Hunger in America

Eating is our most basic need, but in our country, sadly, many people still go hungry each and every day. Many of us think about the large homeless population (over a half a million men, women and children on any given night) when we think of hunger, but unfortunately, chronic hunger impacts far more people than simply those who are homeless.

Food insecurity is a household-level economic and social condition of limited or uncertain access to adequate food.

Hunger is an individual-level physiological condition that may result from food insecurity.

Feeding America in their 2014 study found some startling statistics:

- 1 in 7 Americans lived on incomes that put them at risk for hunger.

- One percent of those requesting emergency food assistance were homeless.

- 42.2 million Americans lived in food insecure households, including 29.1 million adults and 13.1 million children. Food insecurity existed in every single county in the United States.

- 13 percent of households (15.8 million households) were food insecure.

- 5 percent of households (6.3 million households) experienced very low food security.

- Households that had higher rates of food insecurity than the national average included those with children (17%), especially households with children headed by single women (30%) or single men (22%), Black non-Hispanic households (22%) and Hispanic households (19%).

- More than 31 million children lived on incomes that qualify them for free or subsidized lunches.

- Over 15 million American children relied on food banks for assistance.

One important way to Bekindr is to help with this pervasive problem. Many people will give food to people living on the street as a way to practice a random act of kindness. Some will keep food kits in their cars with nonperishable items like granola bars, canned fruit or juices. Perhaps a better way to address food insecurity in your community is by supporting the myriad organizations which address this issue. The largest is Feeding America, a nationwide network of two hundred food banks which leads the fight against hunger in the United States. It provides food to more than 46 million people through sixty thousand food pantries and meal programs in communities across America each year. Feeding America also supports programs that improve food security, educates the public about the problem of hunger, and advocates for legislation that protects people from going hungry.

There are many ways to get involved with this great organization by donating time or money. Many people participate in food drives during the holiday season. Food Banks, however, face their greatest need during the summer months, when classes end and children are no longer receiving free or reduced-cost meals at school, so remember to participate throughout the year.

Thirty-Six Cents
By Robert Murdocco

It was final-exam time in my senior year of college at State University New York Downstate. I had struggled financially throughout the last four years. Money was so tight I often had what I called "hunger anxiety." I was constantly anxious about how I would pay for my next meal. I had come from a middle-class family, but things had fallen apart during my final year of high school when my mom died. My brother and I were left in the care of my stepfather, who provided for us the best he could. We were both in college on scholarships, and we tried to pick up work when we could.

As the end of college approached, I was forced to cut out my part-time jobs in order to have more time to study. Money was so tight I couldn't afford food. Desperately hungry one night, I took a granola bar from my roommate. He noticed and called me out on it. I was filled with shame. That evening, I wandered the campus in search of change. I managed to collect thirty-six cents from the ground, mostly in pennies. I went to the cafeteria, still feeling horrible after the incident with my roommate—and knowing that even with the change I'd found, there was no way I could afford a meal.

Inside, I smelled the food and felt my hunger increase. I looked around, trying to figure out what do. I saw a woman who worked there standing nearby. She looked kind.

I asked her, "Is there a roll or some bread I could get here that costs thirty-six cents?"

She smiled and said, "What do you know! The chicken is on special today, and that's exactly what it costs." She piled a plate high with chicken, rice and vegetables, and I sat down to eat. I felt like I had just won the lottery. She looked like someone who had struggled in her life—like someone who knew just the right thing to do.

Her smile erased my pain. I slept well that night. And I aced my exam the following day.

Then I aced my board exam and I was able to begin my practice as a physical therapist. This allowed me to first support myself and then my family. Although I have never again suffered from hunger anxiety, the events of long ago still impact me. I am disappointed that my roommate and I never reconciled and we lost a friendship over a granola bar, but I feel that the events of that day and night, so long ago, were a turning point in my life. They humbled me in a way that perhaps I needed. I learned what it felt like to be afraid and insecure about making it through the day. This knowledge has helped me in my practice and I am grateful I have found work that allows me to get up every day and help others during their time of need.

"No act of kindness, no matter how small, is ever wasted."

—*Aesop*

The Queen of Hearts

Diana, Princess of Wales, left a truly beautiful legacy. She is recalled most for her grace, style and compassion. She achieved her stated goal, "to be a queen in the hearts of the people."

Princess Diana lived in the pre-Internet era, when the world was not yet flat. She had great concern for anyone who was suffering and shined a spotlight on those in need. She had a passion for helping children and especially those who were ill or injured. She is best remembered for the global attention she brought to those suffering from AIDS, leprosy, homelessness and cancer. She was president or patron of over one hundred charities. She shook everyone's hand and greeted them with her infectious smile. Newspapers called her "the angel of mercy." In June 1997, just one month before her tragic death, she sold 79 of her most expensive dresses at Christie's auction house and raised $3.25 million for charity.

"First, I want to pay tribute to Diana myself. She was an exceptional and gifted human being. In good times and bad, she never lost her capacity to smile and laugh, nor to inspire others with her warmth and kindness. I admired and respected her — for her energy and commitment to others, and especially for her devotion to her two boys."

—*Queen Elizabeth II*

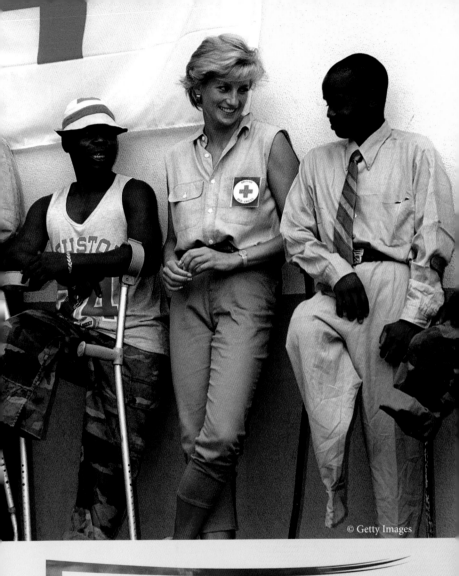

"Carry out a random act of kindness,
with no expectation of reward, safe in
the knowledge that one day someone
might do the same for you."

—*Diana, Princess of Wales*

I Want Them All
By Robert Holmes

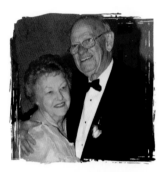

In 1957, with a toolbox and less than $100, I acquired a small avionics shop in exchange for future services. The shop became Aero Systems, Inc. and grew into a multimillion-dollar business based in Miami with operations in London, Paris, California, Hong Kong, Singapore and the Philippines.

My wife, Marjory, and I had two sons, and initially, she was home raising them. In 1959, I asked her to assist in the business on a temporary basis, but she soon became indispensable and remained full-time by my side for the next thirty-five years.

In 1980, we were both working full-time, and we needed some help around the house. We interviewed many women in Miami and couldn't find anyone we liked enough to hire. I was traveling extensively at the time and discussed the situation with an employee in Singapore, who suggested I hire someone from the Philippines. I liked the idea and contacted a friend, Mr. Magallon, a Philippine communications executive, who worked in Manila but lived in a farming town called Santa Barbara on the island of Iloilo. He was a very kind-hearted man whose wife was an elementary school teacher, and together they were always trying to help the young people of their town. On my next trip to the Philippines, Mr. Magallon brought two young women to be interviewed. One of the young women he brought was named Felina. We had an instant chemistry, and I asked her to come to Miami and work with our family.

Felina was twenty-three at the time. She was one of eleven children, and opportunities for her future were quite limited had she remained at home. Felina was frightened when Mr. Magallon brought her to Miami several months later, but she adjusted quickly. Marjory enjoyed teaching her everything around the house—especially cooking.

On my next trip to Manila, I decided to visit Felina's hometown. I met her parents and reassured them that she was in a safe place with a loving family. On my first night there, Mr. Magallon hosted a dinner at his home for Felina's family, her school teachers, classmates and friends as well as several community leaders. It was a wonderful party. I discussed the situation of the people in this small Philippine town with the community leaders, teachers and the young people. There was one fifteen-year-old girl nicknamed Diday who made a big impression on me. She talked my ear off. She wanted so desperately to get an education, to get off the farm and into the bigger world. The next day, Mr. Magallon took me on a tour and showed me the bamboo huts they lived in, and showed me their prize possession: a caribou (a type of cow) which helps them plow the rice fields.

I was very moved by this meeting, by my conversation with Diday, and by the difficult circumstances of this farming town. I wanted to help but realized that giving them money wasn't the answer. I decided that if I could help to educate the children in this community, they could then help themselves and bring their families out of poverty. Marjory and I decided to start a foundation to help these kids get an education. There was free schooling available in Santa Barbara, but many of the kids could not afford the clothes, transportation and books to go to school. They often dropped out to help their parents on the farm. Felina herself had not been able to complete high school.

I told Mr. Magallon of my plan and we set up a group of community leaders to oversee and to operate the foundation. I took a second trip back to Santa Barbara to meet with the local trustees of the Holmes Foundation and to finalize selection of the first group of students. The plan was to select 15 children to become Holmes Scholars. The requirement to become a Holmes Scholar was that the family income had to be less than the equivalent of 2,000 U.S. dollars a year, and the student had to show good academic promise. Mr. Magallon had invited all of the children who had been screened and had met all the qualifications. There were 32 of them. Mr. Magallon announced to the children that the trustees still needed to feed all the information into the computer and then decide which 15 kids would be selected. The scholars would have their clothing, books, lunches and other needs paid as long as they maintained an 85 percent average in school.

When it was my turn to speak, I looked into the eyes of these 32 kids, all so eager to have a chance to excel in life. I simply could not turn down any of them, and so I said, "I want them all."

A large bamboo structure was built in Mr. Magallon's side yard, giving the scholars a special place to meet and to study. Board members supervised the study sessions and were available to help as needed. We communicated through letters with each one of the scholars and traveled to the Philippines twice a year to visit them. We booked several hotel rooms and invited Felina's parents and the scholars to stay in the hotel. They stayed up all night, sang songs, played with the telephone which they had not seen before, and took warm showers. In the morning, the hotel arranged 20 of their dining room tables in a single row, and all the scholars were invited to an American breakfast. I loved seeing their cheerful faces eating eggs and bacon and drinking hot chocolate. It always felt like I received more from the children than I gave.

Seeing the success of the foundation during the first year, we decided we would accept five additional scholars, from fifth grade each year, and offer them an education through college. Neither Marjory nor I had completed college, but we felt strongly that education was the key to improving the lives of these families.

In total, eighty-seven Holmes Scholars have completed a four-year college degree. They were all at the top of their classes, and many became valedictorians and salutatorians. A few went on to graduate school. Most pursued education in areas where they knew they could find work and immigration visas. Nursing and accounting were the most popular.

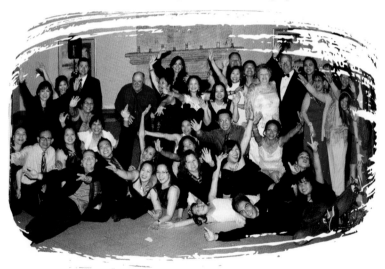

There are now Holmes Scholars scattered around the globe. Twenty-four Holmes scholars are in the U.S. Eight are in Miami working as nurses. Others are in Europe and Saudi Arabia. Some stayed in the Philippines and are making sure the Holmes Foundation carries on. In 1994, Marjory and I retired from business and turned the foundation over to its graduates.

Felina maintains a very special place in our family. In fact, she's my daughter-in-law! Ten years after first arriving, she married our son. They have two boys together. Felina's sister became a Holmes Scholar and now lives in Miami with her husband and two children.

Marjory and I recently celebrated our sixtieth wedding anniversary, and the Holmes Scholars hosted the anniversary party and watched as we renewed our vows. We consider all the scholars to be our children, and we shower them with love. We keep in touch through visits, phone calls and Facebook. Our birthdays, Mother's Day and Father's Day are particularly fun, as we receive greetings from around the world.

Marjory says that the kids taught her to open up her heart. Since she was an only child, this was a very important lesson for her. I have had many accomplishments in my life, but I am most proud of the Holmes Foundation. It is so rewarding to see these kids thriving all over the world. Many are not only providing for themselves but building houses for their parents in the Philippines and sending their siblings to school.

I often marvel at how a simple idea from a friend, ended up helping us, our family and so many families scattered around the globe.

"Unless someone like you cares a whole awful lot, nothing is going to get better. It's not."

—*Dr. Seuss, The Lorax*

The Terminator
By Robert Zuckerman

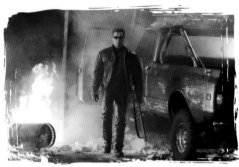

© Robert Zuckerman

In 2002, in Los Angeles, I was the still photographer in the filming of *Terminator 3* with Arnold Schwarzenegger.

One day, between setups, Arnold asked me, "Robert, do you have your cell phone?"

"Sure Arnold," I replied. "I want to talk with your mother!" he said.

So I called my mom in Miami, Florida, happy for this opportunity to add something special to her day. She's been through much in her life and at that time, had two disabled adult daughters under her care.

I put her on the phone with Arnold, and they had a nice conversation for a good five minutes or so. In the end, Arnold told my mom, "Your son is the best photographer I've ever worked with," followed by, "but he doesn't get the credit. *You* do because you produced him!"

I've told this story to many parents over the years because they deserve recognition for their role in the success of their children. My mom is now in a nursing home, but we both still smile as I retell this story to her.

"That's right," she says with her beautiful smile.

Kind Superstars

LeBron James is making headlines not only on the basketball court but also in the rankings of the most generous athletes. In 2015, he pledged $41.8 million to send kids to college in his hometown of Akron, Ohio. Eleven hundred young men and women, who show academic promise, receive four-year college scholarships at the University of Akron. LeBron himself skipped college to join the NBA but he says, "These students have big dreams, and I'm happy to do everything I can to help them get there."

Do Something, a global movement of 5.5 million young people doing good, announced its ninth annual Celebs Gone Good list recognizing the year's celebrities who best use their star power for positive social change. Beyoncé, known as Queen Bey, topped the list for using her platform to highlight a variety of causes including representation of black women in popular culture, the water crisis in Flint, Michigan, gender equality and the Black Lives Matter movement. She also partnered with her husband, Jay-Z, hosting a charity concert to benefit a poverty fighting organization, The Robin Hood Foundation. Together they have created multiple college scholarships for young women who are unafraid to think out of the box. Lin-Manuel Miranda took second place for his participation in the musical tribute "Love Makes the World Go Round," benefitting the victims and the families of the shooting at Pulse, a nightclub in Orlando, Florida.

In June 2016, Born This Way Foundation co-founder Lady Gaga joined philanthropist Phil Anschutz and His Holiness the 14th Dalai Lama to challenge America's cities to be kind. They convened a panel that met in front of more than 200 mayors from across the country and discussed the role that kindness can play in improving the mental health of citizens and how current "cities of kindness" have also experienced a decrease in crime.

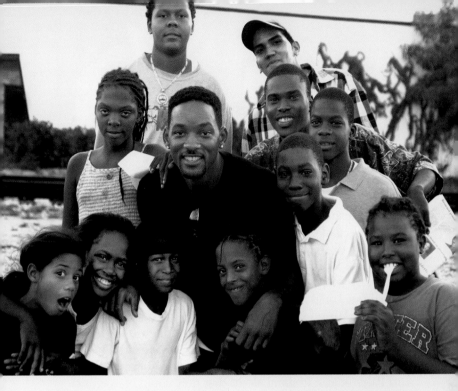

Will Smith during filming of
"Bad Boys 2"

Photo by Robert G. Zuckerman
Copyright © Sony Pictures

"If you're not making someone else's life
better, you're wasting your time."
—Will Smith

Did you know that rock icon Jon Bon Jovi's restaurant,
JBJ Soul Kitchen, in Red Bank, New Jersey, does not have
prices next to the items on its menu? Customers pay with a
conscience—what they can afford. And if they are short on
cash they can earn their meal by working in the kitchen.

Wise Decisions
By Richard Masington

Several years ago, my wife and I were in New York City for a vacation. While there, during one of our many cab rides, we began discussing a plan to engage in direct giving, then we sparked up a conversation with our driver about how his business was doing. He told us he rose at four a.m. to start work at five. He rented his cab, and he usually had to work until about 10:30 a.m. to reach the break-even point, if all went well. His rental payment was more than half of what he could expect to earn in a day. We learned he was a Palestinian immigrant who had lived in New York for years and had family in Palestine. He lamented the state of affairs between Israelis and Palestinians, wishing aloud that they could reason and reconcile with one another. We acknowledged that as Jews, we shared the same feeling.

When we arrived at our destination, we were excited to seize the moment and begin our newly hatched plan. The driver told us the fare, which we gave him. Then we gave him the amount that would cover his cab rental for the day. He was dumbfounded. We exited the cab, and when he had composed himself, he got out as well, so he could give us a hug.

My wife and I were grateful that he gave us this opportunity to give in a way that felt meaningful to all of us. In the years that have elapsed, we have continued to grab these moments, and we feel confident that we are improving the lives of others as we enrich our own.

Airline Seat Lottery
By Anthony Liggins

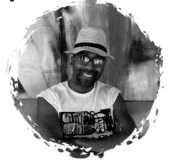

I fly often. I'm an artist, and I travel to see clients, get ideas and visit galleries around the world. Sometimes I catch up on sleep. At other times, I prefer to talk to my seatmate. You never know who it might be. I call it the airline seat lottery.

About three years ago, I was flying from Miami to New York City when I hit the jackpot: I met Pamela Page. Pamela is a filmmaker and had recently been in South Africa shooting a documentary called *No Time for Trouble*. The focus of her film is the power of music to change—and even to save—young lives. It revolves around a poor, but popular, marching band based in Makgofe, a village in northern South Africa.

In Makgofe, boys and girls join gangs as early as the age of ten. By fourteen, they've committed rape, robbery and even murder, part of the growing tide of "gangsterism" that makes this country the most dangerous on the African continent and one of the three most dangerous in the world.

Four years ago, a resident of Makgofe, Janet Bezuidenhout, quit her job, took her life savings and purchased ten musical instruments. She had a simple mission: to keep Makgofe's teenagers off the streets and away from a life of crime. Almost overnight, Bezzi's Youth Brass Band grew in number to sixty girls and boys of all ages and backgrounds.

One by one, with tough love and monetary perks, Janet turns former, current and would-be gang members into drummers and horn players. Lebo plays to forget the mother he's lost. Tumi learns to sew the uniforms to help the band save money. "When Rex decides to stop dealing drugs," Janet says, "We want guys like you."

To keep the village girls safe, she offers them roles as majorettes. Helen has narrowly survived a gang attack, Martha's mother is too poor to replace her daughter's school uniform. Nguaku dreams of a new life in America.

On the plane, Pamela talked passionately about the difficulties of making the film. If not for the generosity of her talented crew, all of whom worked on a deferred basis, she would not have been able to undertake the project. If not for a last-minute introduction to Desmond Tutu's daughter, Pamela would not have had the ability to travel safely in South Africa or capture local gang members on film. If not for the New Orleans musician who is compelled "to go far away and make a difference," the band would not have achieved a new level of competence. If not for a childhood friend who provided funding for additional filming, the project would have died an early death.

I could relate to the film's message: where there's music, there's hope. I grew up in a family that struggled financially. The hardships and challenges Pamela described were familiar terrains. But when I was eight years old, I discovered music, and by the time I was in high school, I had joined the band. I was talented enough to get a scholarship to Delaware State University, where I played in the marching band, as well as the orchestra. I was the first person in my family to attend college. College provided a host of opportunities that changed my life entirely.

Pamela and I talked nonstop on that flight. The three hours literally "flew by." I was so touched listening to her, that when we reached New York, I suggested we exchange contact information.

I've always dreamed of working on a film, and a few weeks after we met, Pamela gave me the chance. She asked me if

I would view her trailer, and assuming I liked what I saw, host a test screening in my Miami gallery. I agreed, and the film, although a work in progress, was every bit as good as I hoped it would be. It was beautiful to watch this impoverished community transformed and uplifted by music.

It was motivating to see how a few shekels, an idea and a dream could inspire people not just locally, but oceans away. I was impressed with the African-American drummer from New Orleans who traveled from afar and infused new energy into the band's fledgling efforts. I will never forget the boy who walked an hour and a half to and from practice every day. When asked why he walked so far, he simply said, "Passion, man. Passion."

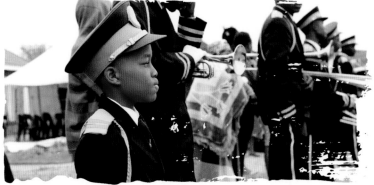

I believe we are at a crossroads, that we are living in an age where kindness and spiritual growth are beginning to take center stage. I believe that in the coming decades, we will all strive to reach a place of greater happiness.

In pursuit of this goal, we should all become messengers for change and use our influence and talent the way Pamela is doing to better humanity. We must all work to unify the cultures around the world. The young and old, the rich and poor, the educated and uneducated must all connect and learn to nourish and support one another. Pamela confirmed to me that extraordinary change is already occurring, and I am so grateful she allowed me to be a part of it.

The Gift
By Pamela Page

From the time I was born until I left for college, my parents traveled, and when they did, a succession of women cooked my meals, stopped my fights, dried my tears, did my laundry and generally taught me the right way to behave.

With Stella, I picked and tasted my first blackberries. From Ginna, I discovered fried plantains, the pleasures of ironing (something I enjoy to this day), and the duty of sharing. From Georgia May, I learned to respect my little brother. From Olivia, who always sang as she worked with a voice every bit as beautiful as Mahalia Jackson's (known as the Queen of Gospel in her time), came a love for the blues and gospel music that has shaped my career to this day.

Olivia made, perhaps, the deepest impression because I was older when she came into our lives via an ad my mother placed in the *Times Picayune*.

Olivia had been working for us for about five years when my parents separated. As an act of protest, my brother and I decided we would not favor one parent over the other with our presence on Thanksgiving Day. The very thought of having to choose so angered us that even if it meant foregoing the gourmet meal that each had planned, we decided to ask Olivia if we could share this holiday with her. Understanding our distress, she offered to host Thanksgiving at her house.

Having never been to Olivia's, we were surprised when we found ourselves driving down a road filled with enormous potholes, just a mile or two from where we lived. We had never considered that all of New Orleans' streets were not perfectly paved like ours was.

Approaching the house, which was little more than a shack, we noticed one of our old sofas on the front porch. Inside the two-room structure was more of our discarded furniture—an old lamp, a small table. A man, who could have been her husband, sat silently on a broken armchair.

Our Thanksgiving dinner was also unexpected. In a flimsy aluminum pan, Olivia had cooked, not a turkey, but what appeared to be a gigantic rat. Seeing our surprise, she asked, "So you never ate possum before?"

"No. Never."

Yet in the company of dear, kind Olivia, far from my warring parents, crowded around our ex-table, this humble meal tasted better to me than any Thanksgiving feast before or since.

That year, my father gave me a car. I could now explore the city, and the parts of New Orleans that interested me most were the musical ones, so I asked Olivia if I could visit her church. I knew her choir was making a record, and I wanted to hear them sing. It didn't occur to me that I would be the only white person there, nor did I suspect that I would have to introduce myself to the entire congregation. Being in the spotlight has always terrified me, but there I was, in front of a few hundred mostly older people. When the service ended, many of Olivia's friends introduced themselves, told me how nice I looked and that they hoped to see me the following Sunday. I don't know who was prouder that day—me for standing up and saying my name, or Olivia for showing off her new congregant.

My last memory of Olivia was at my high school graduation. As far as I was concerned, Olivia was family. It was therefore natural that she should share this important occasion with us. I remember looking out at the crowd of parents, grandparents, brothers and sisters and seeing Olivia dressed in her finest, the only African-American present, standing at the back of the group beaming up at me.

I left for an internship in Washington, D.C. soon after and went on to begin a career as a filmmaker in New York. My specialty is music; my passion is black culture—the gift of my earliest mentors.

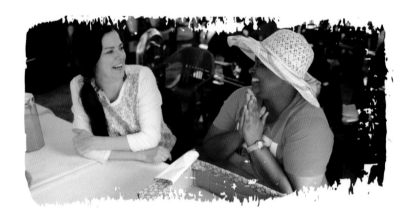

"Life's most persistent and nagging question is what are you doing for others."

—*Martin Luther King, Jr.*

Lessons From Nelson Mandela

Rick Stengel spent the better part of two years working with Nelson Mandela on his autobiography, *Long Walk to Freedom*. Here's what Stengel told Time Magazine: "In 1994, during the presidential-election campaign, Mandela got on a tiny propeller plane to fly down to the killing fields of Natal and give a speech to his Zulu supporters. I agreed to meet him at the airport, where we would continue our work after his speech. When the plane was 20 minutes from landing, one of its engines failed. Some on the plane began to panic. The only thing that calmed them was looking at Mandela, who quietly read his newspaper, as if he were a commuter on his morning train to the office. The airport prepared for an emergency landing, and the pilot managed to land the plane safely. When Mandela and I got in the backseat of his bulletproof BMW that would take us to the rally, he turned to me and said, 'Man, I was terrified up there!'"

You can see from this story, Mr. Mandela was able to remain calm in even the most life-threatening situation. According to his biography, he used his 27 years in jail to meditate and contemplate his own mind and feelings and emerged with a deep and overflowing love for all of humanity. Regular meditation strengthens our vagal tone and he recommends 15 minutes before bedtime. Enhanced vagal tone increases our parasympathetic response ("tend and befriend") which counteracts our sympathetic response ("fight or flight"). While I hope our readers are never faced with such a grave challenge, increasing your vagal tone will benefit you when dealing with more mundane stresses that we all face, such as time urgency and driving in traffic.

This One's on Me
By Danielle Castellanos

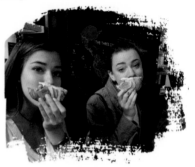

It was the first time I decided to visit my father's grave alone, and I was flooded with emotions. I drove my car to the neighborhood we grew up in and decided to stop at Einstein's bagel shop; the one where my dad and I had our last breakfast together. The shop held nothing but good memories, but still, I was sad replaying them all in my mind. I ordered an "everything" bagel with cream cheese, Dad's favorite, and took my seat to wait patiently.

The customer ahead of me gave the cashier a hard time about something trivial and walked out in a huff. Then the cashier looked over at me and apologized for the commotion. "This one's on me," he said as he handed me my breakfast. I smiled for the first time that day, and my mood lifted instantly. He'll never know it, but that simple gesture from a kind stranger felt like a gift from my dad himself, and it got me through that tough first visit without tears.

"The shortest distance between two people is a smile."

—Victor Borge

We Can be Heroes
By Nancy Zaretsky

One afternoon not long ago, I was walking along the beach in Bal Harbour, catching up with a friend on the phone. It's a beautiful path and one that people from around the world travel to Florida to enjoy. As I came up to the jetty at Haulover Inlet, I noticed an older woman with a little girl in a black baby stroller. The woman's back was turned to the stroller, as she looked at the buildings in the distance.

In an instant, the stroller started to roll toward the edge of the jetty.

To my left, a blonde woman in a black top began shouting, "The stroller, the stroller!" as she ran toward the jetty. The older

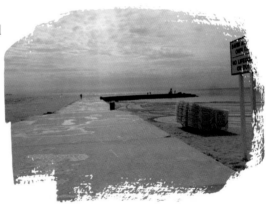

woman had no idea the stroller was moving. As I ran toward the edge, I told my friend I had to call 911. The stroller went over the edge and into the inlet. The blonde woman jumped over the edge after it, and I dropped my phone, realizing there was no time for 911.

I watched the blonde woman down on the rocks as she clutched the stroller handle, fighting the waves and unbuckling the baby girl. Both had been bloodied by the barnacles and rocks. The current was sucking the stroller into the inlet; it was a battle between the sea and the blonde woman who was determined to rescue the infant. I grabbed the stroller and helped the woman pass the baby to a young man who had come to help. We passed the baby up, grabbed the submerged stroller, and took turns heading back up the rocks.

Once over the top, the blonde woman and I cried and hugged each other for a long time. The woman with the stroller comforted the baby, together with another passerby. I don't know the names of the brave woman who jumped over the edge so quickly or the man who brought the baby to the top. But I do know that they are the kind of people I think of when I think of the extraordinary people who populate my city, my country, this world.

"Next to creating a life the finest thing a man can do is save one."

—Abraham Lincoln

Kindness Today

There is nothing new about the idea of being kind. The word kindness is mentioned over one hundred times in the Bible. One of the older definitions of the word kind in the Oxford English Dictionary reads: "To act according to one's nature…The manner or way natural or proper to anyone."

Many people are remembered throughout history for their extraordinary kindness, including Jesus, Nelson Mandela, Dr. Martin Luther King, Jr., His Holiness the Dalai Lama and Buddha, to name just a few. The Underground Railroad, which stretched from the slave states into the free states and Canada, was composed of a chain of volunteers who freed 100,000 slaves by 1850. The Underground Railroad was, in fact, neither. It was a series of meeting points, secret routes, transportation and safe houses operated by a long string of strangers, and it may serve as one of history's best examples of the powerful ability of the kindness of strangers to change the world.

What is new is that we may be confused about how to be kind in our ultra-connected, driven world. Social media has made our relationships so complicated that our innate drive to be kind can easily get lost in the noise. We must make an effort to Bekindr.

There is a movement underway to spread kindness, and examples abound. Google searches for the word kindness doubled in 2016. The ball that dropped in Times Square ushering in 2017, watched by one billion people, was composed of kindness triangles made of Waterford Crystal introducing the Gift of Kindness design. The inspiring Broadway musical, *Come From Away*, which recounts the story of the planes landing in Newfoundland on 9/11, celebrates the kindness of strangers and opened to rave reviews and won a Tony Award®. College admissions boards around the country are following the lead of

Harvard University and selecting students who show kindness instead of overachieving. Harvard Graduate School of Education released a report in January 2016 entitled, *Turning the Tide: Inspiring Concern for Others and the Common Good Through College Admissions*. There was a recent *NY Times* Opinion Section piece about a student unanimously selected for admission by the Dartmouth admissions committee because he included a letter of reference from his high school custodian, who lauded the student for this thoughtfulness.

Do you know when the best time is to plant an oak tree? Twenty years ago. Do you know the second-best time? Now! So now is the time to plant more kindness.

© Kate Luber

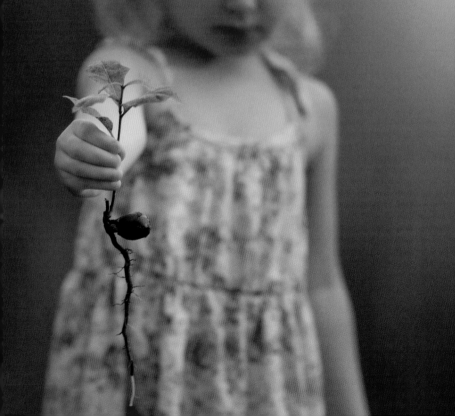

Two Angels in Austria
By Barbara Bibas Montero

On July 21, 2013, my husband and I checked into a hotel in Vienna, Austria, after having attended a lovely wedding at a castle outside the city. Around 7 p.m., I heard my husband gasping for air. He soon lost consciousness. I frantically began administering CPR, and then, realizing I needed help, telephoned downstairs asking reception to call an ambulance. Within minutes, two employees came to the room with special equipment and, thankfully, paramedics arrived minutes later. They were able to stabilize my husband's weak pulse after many attempts with the defibrillator. He had suffered an arrhythmia.

The manager on duty, Anton, and the Director of Sales, Anna, were the two employees who had come to my rescue. Seeing that I was distraught, they helped with everything from the language translation with the paramedics to making sure I had a glass of water. They held my hand as I cried and cried.

When the paramedics took my husband downstairs on a stretcher, I tried to go with him to the hospital, but they would not allow me to ride in the ambulance. I found out later that the paramedics were not sure my husband was going to make it, and they hadn't wanted me to be in the vehicle, in case the worst happened. Anton and Anna drove me to the hospital themselves, comforting me the whole way there. The situation filled me with both terror and disbelief. We had come here for a wedding, a joyful occasion, and now my husband might never leave. I struggled to understand how it was possible.

For two hours, Anna and Anton stayed with me at the hospital, communicating with the doctors, translating important information. Once my husband was stabilized in the ICU, they drove me back to the hotel.

My husband stayed in a coma for two weeks. Every day we would visit him for the couple of hours we were allowed to do so, and during this trying time, both Anton and Anna were like two angels. They rallied their staff to assist my daughters, who had flown in from the United States and were willing to do anything possible to make us feel at home. Special snacks and sweets were left in our room every evening; heartfelt notes and ceramic angels were left on our pillows. The outpouring of kindness, love and hope was humbling.

My dear husband never woke up—he died on August 5th. I was overcome with grief—stuck in a strange land, with nearly everyone I knew thousands of miles and time zones away. My daughters and I clung to each other, heartbroken. It was a sad day for all of us. Anton and Anna were there throughout, comforting us and trying to ease our pain. When it was time to return home, they invited us to dinner the evening before our departure and presented us with bracelets inscribed with uplifting messages. Although the circumstances were tragic, we will never forget Anton and Anna and the extraordinary kindness we received.

"There are no strangers here; only friends you haven't yet met."
—*William Butler Yeats*

Converse?
By Rob Polishook

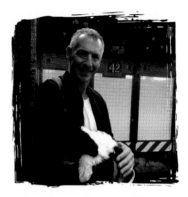

It was 10:00 p.m., and I was returning from dinner with a friend. We had a great time, caught up on each other's lives and ate some delicious food! At the end of the evening, I was the beneficiary of a leftover lamb burger with cheese. I anticipated having this burger for tomorrow's lunch—that was until I saw a shoeless man walk onto the subway. At first, I admit, I saw him and then walked down to another car. From a distance, I noticed a young woman talking to him. He was very calm as they chatted. The woman continued to talk with him and I decided to inch closer.

I moved opposite them and saw his swollen feet. I quickly assessed my white converse sneakers and thought about giving them to him, but realized they simply would not fit. I then decided tomorrow's lunch was no longer important to me—he could use it much more. As the subway arrived at my stop, I handed it to him. I saw him take his first bite of the sandwich. It was clear he enjoyed it!

You're My Hero
By Mariana Cruz

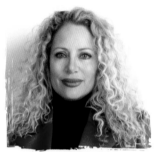

© Robert Zuckerman

I first saw Major Ed Pulido, U.S. Army (Ret.), in 2014, as he stood on a stage in Florida, and described how he and his friends had raised $250,000 to pay for his titanium leg after he was hit by a roadside bomb in Iraq. He spoke about life after combat with the purpose of giving a voice to other veterans.

One of the veterans with him was SSG Mike Harryman, U.S. Army (Ret.), a sniper who had fought in Afghanistan and Iraq. He was wounded multiple times and received four Purple Hearts and a Bronze Star for his service. Though Mike didn't speak that night, I sought him out to hear his story; I was interested to know what his daily life was like now that he had returned home. I knew that when these brave men and women return home from war, they often struggle to reintegrate back into the society they fought for.

Twenty-two American veterans commit suicide every day, and one of the main reasons is social isolation. My father was a Marine, so I was raised to appreciate the sacrifices of our military. Still, I can't even imagine what life is like for soldiers dealing with PTSD, depression, multiple medical issues, the complex Veteran's Administration system, financial issues, and the struggle of finding employment after the military, on top of all life's usual difficulties and uncertainties.

I was able to track Mike down, and I began calling him

every few days to check in. These phone calls became the starting point of our friendship. Mike had served three tours of duty—one in Afghanistan, and two in Iraq. Though he was wounded multiple times, he kept reenlisting. When I asked him why, he said he wanted to provide a better life for his newborn daughter and wife. However, his final combat injury would change his life forever. Mike was hit in the face with a .57mm anti-armor rocket and was pronounced dead on the side of a dirt road in Iraq.

Fifteen days later, this highly trained Army sniper woke from a coma in Walter Reed Hospital and tried to kill the nurse, thinking he had been captured.

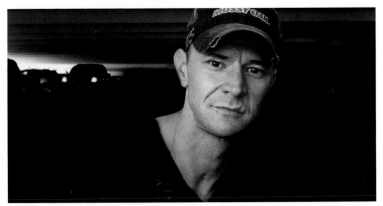

© Robert Zuckerman

The lower half of his face had been blown off, his teeth were knocked out, he had lost half his tongue and suffered a traumatic brain injury. He was in the hospital for so long and was given so much pain medicine that he became addicted. When he was finally able to go home, Mike found his marriage in shambles. He was an addict.

His doctors would no longer give him the drugs upon which he was now dependent, so he turned to the streets.

By the time I met Mike, he had been divorced twice. He was

now in recovery and attending church in Oklahoma City. He was in his early thirties.

One day I asked Mike, "If you could meet anyone in the world, who would you want to meet?"

He answered, "Joyce Meyer. I used to watch her every day on TV when I was recovering in the hospital. And Dwayne "The Rock" Johnson because he's one of my heroes."

I smiled and said, "I can make that happen." It just so happened that I had recently met Joyce Meyer through my minister Robyn Wilkerson and knew she would be speaking at Trinity Church in two months. Mike's dream of meeting Joyce Meyer came true in Miami and then again in Oklahoma, where Mike invited other veterans to meet Joyce and her husband, Dave, at their conference.

I wanted to do something more for Mike, and I had an idea about giving a group of veterans a voice so people could appreciate their sacrifices. I planned to go to Oklahoma City and hire a camera crew to film a gathering for veterans that Mike was participating in. I flew to Oklahoma, checked into

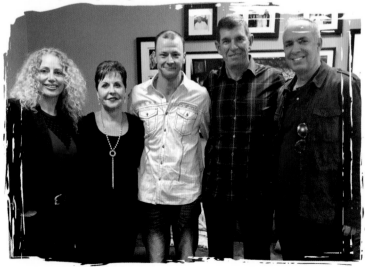

a hotel and got to know a group of amazing men and women. When I heard their stories, I was often speechless at their bravery, at the personal toll they had each paid for our country. I would say, "You're a hero!" And they would shake their heads and say, "The real heroes came home in coffins."

This diverse group of veterans I met in Oklahoma was incredible. When I returned to Miami and told friends

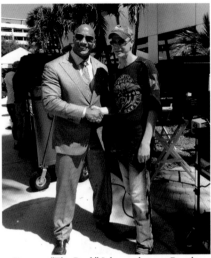

Dwayne "The Rock" Johnson honors Purple Heart Recipient SSG Mike Harryman, U.S. Army (Ret.) on the set of HBO's Ballers.

about the heroes I had met, they wanted to meet them too. So we invited Mike to stay with our family. He had never been to Miami. He gave me a list of things he wanted to do: jump in the Atlantic Ocean, see a Lamborghini, visit the Everglades. My husband and I greeted Mike at the airport and set out to do every last thing on his list. And a curious thing happened: Kindness proliferated throughout his visit. Dwayne Johnson invited Mike to the set of HBO's *Ballers*. Mike was also invited to go boating and to dinner parties as the honored guest. Our kids became close to him and loved listening to his stories.

At one point during his visit, Mike turned to me and said, "Mariana, you're my hero." It was one of the most meaningful moments of my life. I had started out wanting to give something to Mike, to thank him for his service, and he ended up giving me much more.

Ways to Bekindr

Behavioral change takes time, but our brains are designed to change. Scientists call this phenomenon "neuroplasticity." We now know you can teach an old dog a new trick, but it's still easier to train a puppy (under twenty-five in people years). Repetition is the key to forming new pathways in the brain and modifying the way you think, act and feel. The Oxford dictionary defines kindness as "The quality of being friendly, generous and considerate." Sounds simple and wise! I believe that being kind is an essential ingredient to becoming a citizen in good standing in your community and our world. I am guessing that since you are reading this book, you do too!

Kindness should start with you. Each of us has a responsibility to treat ourselves in a kind fashion. By this, I mean things that sound simple but can be quite challenging such as engaging in positive self-talk. Often we don't even recognize that we are not being kind to ourselves. We may have constant negative chatter in our head, and we might need to acknowledge, and then change that aspect of our daily life.

Take good care of yourself. Rest properly. (Sleep is the base of the wellness pyramid. It's hard to do anything right when you are exhausted.) Nourish yourself, and avoid toxins like excess stress, drugs or misuse of alcohol. We may be drinking too much and feeling depressed the next day and not realizing these events are connected. We may be so used to stress that we forget there is a more positive way to live. Exercise regularly. Walk. We must be kind to ourselves first and foremost. Everything begins within, and can then be projected into the world.

We can also practice being kind to those closest to us: our family, our loved ones and our dearest friends. Ways to improve these relationships abound. We can also work on being kinder to acquaintances who may or may not one day become friends. We can Bekindr to our environment, which needs us now more than ever. We can be kind to animals in a variety of ways, from nurturing them as pets to choosing to eat less meat. And finally, we can choose to work on kindness to strangers, the subject of this book.

Here's a list of kind behaviors to help you generate ways to Bekindr.

To yourself:

- Make sure your self-talk is positive.
- Go to bed early.
- Eat healthy snacks.
- Give yourself a digital detox.
- Book a massage.
- Take a bath or shower.
- Practice meditation or deep breathing.
- Listen to a relaxation tape.
- Schedule a doctor or dentist visit.
- Do the chore or errand you have been putting off.
- Avoid electronic devices one or two hours before bedtime.
- Skip reading or watching any news for one day.
- Drink more water.
- Make sure you get up every forty-five minutes when you are sitting.
- Take a walk.
- Spend time in nature.
- Make time to work out.
- Drink a cup of tea.
- Read an inspiring book.
- Make time to laugh.
- Listen to music.
- Journal.
- Talk to your doctor about brain health.
- Work on reducing your stress level.
- Avoid rushing.
- Sign up for an app or website that sends you inspirational or funny messages daily.
- Learn something new.
- Listen to a TED talk or Podcast.
- Nourish your spiritual or religious side by attending a religious ceremony or lecture or spend time in prayer or contemplation.

To loved ones and friends:

- Smile!
- Make eye contact.
- Call instead of texting.
- Hold someone's hand.
- Listen attentively.
- Send a handwritten note.
- Put your phone away when speaking to someone.
- Visit a friend.
- Offer to run errands with someone or do a chore for them.
- Help someone clean up or organize his or her home or office.
- Say "I love you."
- Help someone with a chore.
- Write something nice to someone on social media.
- Offer to help a friend who is moving or under stress.
- Cook for someone.
- Bring food to work to share.
- Reach out to a friend you haven't spoken to for a while.
- Give someone flowers.
- Share inspirational quotes and humor.
- Buy someone coffee or lunch.
- Frame a picture of someone and send it to them.
- Bring someone breakfast in bed.
- Hug!
- Ask a friend to join you for a workout.
- Teach someone something.
- Bring the neighbor's trash can back in or remove snow or leaves from the driveway.
- Give someone a heartfelt compliment.
- Hand something down to someone.
- Give someone a gift.
- Make someone a playlist.
- Donate time or money to a charity that is important to a friend or loved one.
- Express gratitude.

To strangers:

- Smile!
- Make sure you say "please" and "thank you."
- Let someone go in front of you in traffic or in a line.
- Respect crosswalks.
- Hold a door open.
- Help someone carry something.
- Offer to take someone's picture.
- Ask the cashier/waiter/receptionist/doorman/valet how their day is going.
- Pay for someone behind you in line at a coffee shop or toll plaza.
- Give food/money/clothing to someone who is homeless.
- Over tip.
- Give someone a compliment.
- Write a thank you note to your trash collector, mailman, firemen or policemen.
- Donate money to a charity.
- Volunteer!

To animals:

- Give your pet some extra attention.
- Adopt a pet.
- Pay the pet adoption fee for someone else to adopt an animal from a shelter.
- Buy humanely raised products.
- Reduce your meat and dairy intake.
- Take your pet to the vet.
- Send money to organizations that support animals like the Humane Society of the U.S.
- Volunteer at a local animal shelter.

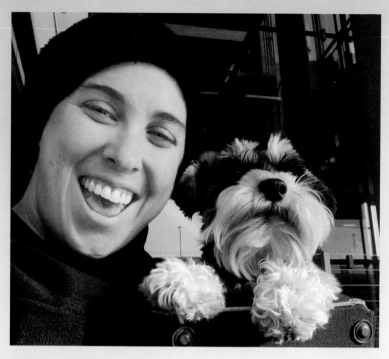

To the environment:

- Turn your lights off.
- Avoid plastic!
- Dress for the weather indoors instead of raising the air conditioner or heat.
- Recycle.
- Pick up trash.
- Walk instead of driving.
- Share a Lyft, Uber, Gett, Juno or Via ride.
- Use public transportation.
- Carpool.
- Eat leftovers and avoid food waste.
- Plant a garden.
- Carry your own mug to a coffee shop, most will give you a discount.
- Buy locally grown food.
- Bring your own bag to the store.
- Choose used when buying books, clothes and other items.
- Buy a BPA-free bottle for water and refill often.
- Avoid paper when possible.
- Switch to LED lighting.
- Shut off the water when you are brushing your teeth.

I Have Daughters, Too
By Sue Ann Greenfield

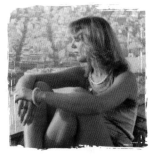

In 1977, I was living in a tiny studio apartment in New York
City, working as a legal secretary and dreaming of my first
solo trip to Greece. I was twenty years old. When my shiny new
American Express card arrived, I was finally on my way.

On my flight from Kennedy Airport to Athens, I met a girl
named Susan. She had been to Greece before and was going
again to meet up with friends. She asked me to join her "tribe"
when we arrived in Mykonos. When we landed, we parted
ways and agreed to meet for dinner the following evening.

I arrived at my hotel outside of town and was stunned by
how beautiful it was. What a view of the Mediterranean! I was
in heaven. After a few hours and a beer enjoyed by the sea, I
left to meet Susan in the village. That night, over dinner, we
decided to take a day trip to Hydra—a small, charming island
nearby—the next day.

I traveled light with a knapsack containing my passport, hotel
key, money, a change of clothes and a small lunch. I carefully
placed the knapsack in a locker during the one-hour boat ride
over. When we arrived, we headed toward the beach to soak up
the sun and enjoy each other's company.

After many hours of fun, we began to make our way back
to the boat. We suddenly realized it had grown quite late and
began to rush, a bit worried that we might miss the last boat off

the island. We waited for the commuter bus to the pier…which never came. Few on Hydra spoke English, and because the island was at the time not well populated by tourists, Susan and I found ourselves surrounded by locals with whom we could not communicate.

The bus finally came, and we knew we were cutting it close. Sure enough, when we finally arrived back at the dock, the boat had left without us. I remember thinking, maybe this vacation wasn't a good idea.

Fighting tears, we waited and waited, until finally, a fishing boat full of men arrived at the dock. It smelled awful! The fishermen were dirty and sweaty from a day's work. They didn't speak a word of English. Somehow, though, we figured out that they were going back to the port from which we had left. We climbed aboard and stuck close by each other for the duration of the trip.

When we finally arrived at the port, it was dark and cold. We were exhausted, disheveled and hungry—but the kindness of the fishermen had been so heartwarming that we hardly noticed our discomfort. They smiled and waved goodbye. They had known we were in trouble and had helped us so generously.

But the real kindness came when we got off their boat and encountered a man sitting beside the dock—one of the attendants who had helped us stow our luggage on our initial boat ride. As we approached him, I saw that he was holding my knapsack in his hand. He had waited for us for many hours, hoping we would return. I hugged and thanked him, and he said the four words I've never forgotten in the years since: "I have daughters, too."

Cell Phones and Kindness

Researchers from Kent State's College of Education, Health and Human Services surveyed 493 students, ranging in age from eighteen to twenty-nine, to look at the effect of cell phone use on social connectedness.

In 2016, they reported female students spend an average of 365 minutes per day on their cell phones, sending and receiving an average of 265 texts per day, and making and receiving six calls per day.

Male students reported spending less time on their phones (287 minutes), sending and receiving fewer texts (190), and making and receiving the same number of calls as the female students.

For the women, the study found that talking on the phone was associated with feeling emotionally close to their parents and friends. For the men, the opposite was true—daily calling and texting were not related in any way to feelings of emotional closeness with either parents or peers.

What surprised me most about this study is the amount of time both sexes are spending on their phones. Six hours a day for women and almost five hours a day for men!

On average, people in the United States across all age groups check their phones forty-six times per day, according to Deloitte, one of the "Big Four" accounting firms, in 2015. That's up from thirty-three looks per day in 2014.

Although forty-six checks per day is the average, that number varies according to the user's age group. Those between the ages of eighteen and twenty-four look at their phones most often, with an average of seventy-four checks per day. Americans in the twenty-five to thirty-four age bracket look at their devices fifty times per day, and those between thirty-five and forty-four do so thirty-five times each day.

Deloitte also found that 81 percent of Americans spend time looking at their phones while dining out in restaurants. Arianna Huffington says, "Getting rid of technology seems to be the next frontier in table manners."

Most respondents across all age groups said they look at their phones within five minutes of waking up. Twenty-six percent of those in the eighteen to twenty-four age range said they look at their phones immediately upon waking up.

So what does this all have to do with kindness?

Dr. Sara Konrath at the University of Michigan has been assessing empathy and compassion, and she has come up with some alarming results. In reviewing a standard assessment of empathy and compassion taken by thirteen thousand college students between 1979 and 2009, Dr. Konrath discovered that self-reported concern for the welfare of others has been steadily dropping since the early 1990s. According to this analysis, levels of compassion and empathy are lower now than at any time in the past thirty years. Perhaps most alarming, they are declining at an increasing rate. She postulates that our cell phone obsession is contributing to our declining scores. Readers, please note that her research was done in 2009. I think we all know which direction cell phone use has gone in the subsequent years!

Time spent on cell phones is time not spent in face-to-face interaction. We don't trigger our mirror neurons and our capacity to be empathic is greatly reduced. We are having a far greater number of brief, often superficial conversations with a much larger number of people, and as a result, we are losing our ability to connect in deep and meaningful ways.

One simple way to Bekindr is to put down your cell phone and connect to those right in front of you. It may sound old-fashioned, but it makes a lot of sense. It's what our brains are designed to do. Start by not inviting your cell phone to meals, and see if you can get your friends to do the same.

What Really Matters
By Gordon Hurd

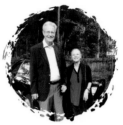

On September 5, 1991, I returned home from an extensive stay in a hospital in Germany. I had entered the hospital on July 19th with what was diagnosed as a gallstone. After initial surgery and the removal of a one-inch stone, there were major complications, which resulted in five additional surgeries and my being placed on a life-support system in the intensive-care ward for more than two weeks. I came out of the coma on August 15th, and I remained hospitalized for an additional two weeks as I gained strength and some of the fifty-five pounds I had lost.

When I was sent home, I had a fifteen-inch open wound that had to be treated on a daily basis. My family physician came by every evening upon completing his hospital and office practice and attended to my wound. During my recovery, I had very little strength and was often in pain from the multiple surgeries.

One particularly bad day, while the doctor was tending my wound, I complained to him about my situation. Although my physician was German and we spoke in a combination of German and English, we understood what each of us meant even if we didn't translate word for word. His words to me then have formed the basis for the rest of my life. He told me that I had to make a decision *now*—to either feel sorry for myself because of what I had gone through or to recognize that I had been held to this earth by the tiniest of threads. He told me that I should always remember what really mattered to me in life—my family and those who cared about me—like he did. It was a moment that I have never forgotten, and I can recall that conversation (which occurred over twenty-five years ago) as if it was yesterday.

Too Much Kindness?

My seventeen-year-old nephew saw a blood drive at his school, so he went in to donate. Since he was a minor, they called my sister to ask permission, and she said "Yes." A few minutes later he texted her and said his blood count was very high, and they wanted to take two units. My sister was working and didn't see the message. Twenty minutes later she replied "No." He texted back, "Too late." A few hours later, she watched him try to play at an important high school baseball game, and he was so weak he could barely stand. That was clearly one pint of kindness too much!

It is not uncommon for couples or family members to disagree about the right amount of kindness. Should you spend the holiday feeding people who are in shelters, or should you host your own family? Should you donate your raise to the local children's hospital, or take your family on vacation? Is it safe to send your teenage daughter to volunteer at a food kitchen? Should you adopt a child? Should you miss a week of work to volunteer for Habitat for Humanity? These are very complex matters and require candid discussions to make sure everyone is on the same page. Acts of kindness can take you away from your family and many require family support. It is important to consider those nearest to us, and carefully evaluate their opinions when deciding how much and what type of kindness is right for you and your family.

"Without the human community, one single human being cannot survive."
—His Holiness the Dalai Lama

The Gift of Life
By Marc Hurwitz

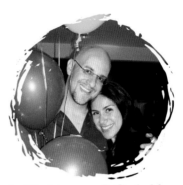

In the late 1990s, my synagogue in Washington, D.C., held a blood drive. As I was donating, the nurse asked me if I would agree to have my cheek swabbed for the national bone marrow registry. I said yes.

Nearly a decade later, in 2009, I received a phone call.

That hadn't been an easy year for me. I had recently left my long-term government job and was struggling financially. I was only working on a few small contracts, trying to build my own business. My fiancée and I were preparing to move into a less expensive apartment in order to get by.

The call came on a weekday afternoon. I was informed that I might be a possible match for someone in need of bone-marrow stem cells—an outcome whose probability is one in millions. Immediately, I was filled with excitement; it never crossed my mind to say no. I saw only one option, and that was to move forward with the process, whatever it might entail.

That brief phone call set off a whirlwind of activity, resulting in an experience that would change me forever. I met with the local community blood center on several occasions for additional testing. A nurse came to our apartment a few times to take more blood samples—twenty-four tubes, at one point. After the tests were finished, I was told not to take any risks with my life—no skydiving, for example. The recipient had been taken off crucial life-saving protocols to prepare for the stem-cell infusion, which meant that there was no turning back. She now needed my stem cells more than ever.

The donor process involved three concurrent days of blood dialysis: blood being taken out of one arm, "washed" in a machine that extracted the bone marrow stem cells and then reinjected into my other arm. During the three days, and for several weeks after, I endured the expected side effects: bone aches, especially in my back. At the end of the third day, my fiancée and I watched as the stem cells were packed into a shipping cooler to be taken straight to the airport, en route to an anonymous female recipient in England. Due to privacy laws there, the recipient and I were not allowed to know each other. We wrote a letter that we hoped would reach her; we never heard back. To this day, we don't know if she survived.

Still, this may be for the best. We are taught in the Jewish tradition that the highest form of *tzedakah*, or charity, is to give without knowing the recipient.

As I was recovering from my bone aches, my wonderful fiancée threw me a surprise party to acknowledge my gift. She rented out a restaurant and filled it with my friends. It was touching and reinforced what I already knew to be true—that she's an amazing woman with a huge heart. Her encouragement and support through the process gave me strength and helped us fall even deeper in love.

During my recovery, as we were moving to a new apartment, I became sick as a result of a lowered immune system from the process, and it took me almost a month to fully recover. I had never been sick for so long. Yet looking back, I am filled with so much warmth thinking about the whole experience.

We all strive to find meaning in our lives. This could be yours. You have the power to potentially save a life. Knowing that I helped someone in that way means everything to me.

Kindness and the Web

Jonathan L. Zittrain, a professor at Harvard Law School, in his compelling TED talk, "Web as Random Acts of Kindness" describes the Internet in a very optimistic way. According to Zittrain, the Web is a remarkable creation of individuals, many of whom volunteer their time to pass on information the way we might pass the beer down the row at a sporting event.

Professor Zittrain uses the example of Wikipedia, the free-access Internet encyclopedia that is entirely created, updated and monitored by volunteers. Wikipedia is the largest and most popular general reference work on the Internet, launched in 2001, consisting of more than 40 million articles in over 250 different languages. It is the sixth most visited website in the U.S. behind Google, Facebook, YouTube, Yahoo and Amazon. As Sir Francis Bacon said in 1597, "Knowledge is power," and indeed that is true. The Internet has created an explosion of information unlike anything before it.

Similarly, Khan Academy (khanacademy.org), a nonprofit created in 2006 by educator Salman Khan, provides a free, world-class education for anyone, anywhere. The organization produces short lectures in the form of YouTube videos and supplementary practice exercises and tools for educators. The website and its content are provided mainly in English but are also available in other languages like Bengali, Hindi and Spanish. The academy started organically, when Salman Khan was tutoring one of his cousins on the Internet. Other cousins heard about it and wanted to join in. The website is now a global movement, with over 10 million unique visitors a month and millions of dollars pouring in from the Bill and Melinda Gates Foundation, Google and many more. What could be kinder than providing a free education to everyone?

Almost every aspect of our life has been changed by the Internet. Waze, a community-oriented GPS app, allows users to submit road information and route data based on location, such as reports of car accidents or traffic and integrates that data into its routing algorithms for all users of the app thus making one of our biggest stressors just a bit more tolerable. That is kind to drivers and our environment.

You might not think of kindness immediately when you think of Lyft/Uber and Airbnb/VRBO (Vacation Rentals by Owner) but I urge you to think again. People are opening their most valuable assets, cars and homes, letting strangers into places typically reserved for close friends and family. These companies are revolutionizing the way we move around and without kindness, they will cease to exist. We are social creatures, and when our urge to connect can be monetized it creates a powerful win-win situation.

The Internet has greatly impacted the flow of money and makes kindness through donations easier and smarter than ever. JustGiving (justgiving.com), established in 2001, allows the public to help raise money for charities and has become the most popular platform for online giving in the world. Their mission is to ensure no great cause goes unfunded. They have helped people in 164 countries raise over $4.2 billion for good causes since their inception. That sounds pretty kind to me! GoFundMe is a crowdfunding platform that allows people in a number of countries to raise money for events ranging from celebrations and graduations to challenging circumstances like accidents and illnesses. The company has raised over 3 billion dollars since its inception in 2010.

The Internet even facilitates giving of yourself. Marc Hurwitz shared his story of donating his bone marrow through Be the Match®, operated by the National Marrow Donor Program® (NMDP). They are the world's largest registry, with more than 27 million potential donors. The National Kidney

Registry has 50,000 living potential kidney donors enrolled. These kind donors take giving of themselves to the highest level.

For those who wish to donate organs after their death, enrolling is easy. Simply sign up online at dmv.org or organdonor.gov or in person at the Department of Motor Vehicles. Register, and join the other 100 million registered organ donors in the United States. There are more than 120,000 Americans awaiting their organ transplants, and a single organ donor has the potential to save up to eight lives.

"A human being is a part of the whole called by us "Universe"...Our task must be to free ourselves...by widening our circle of compassion to embrace all living creatures and the whole of nature in its beauty."

—Albert Einstein

Welcome Home
By O. Toki

I first came to the United States in the summer of 1980. I was a high school exchange student from Japan, on the first foreign trip of my life. As a matter of fact, it was the first foreign trip ever taken by anyone in my immediate family. Not unusual, really—the focus in Japan was always on schooling for the children and work for the adults. Anything else was considered frivolous.

We weren't well off—far from it—but were financially secure, thanks to Japan's lifetime employment system. And both my older brother and I attended one of the top boys' prep schools, one with a well-established history of sending its graduates to top universities. In education-focused Japan, this school's name carried a tremendous amount of weight.

Yet I was beginning to feel constrained by the complicated ways of Japanese society. To me, so much of it seemed unnecessary, even irrational. Particularly in comparison to how things worked in the U.S.—at least as far as I understood it based on newspapers, books, films and television. That nagging feeling only grew, eventually leading me to participate in a one-year exchange student program to see the U.S. for myself. If I liked it, I would try to emigrate. The stakes were real: I understood, without a doubt, that opting out of the Japanese education system this way, even temporarily, would put a permanent question mark on my record. If I ended up coming back to Japan, I wouldn't be able to simply get back on the "elite" path I was on. But I was willing to risk it. To their credit, my parents supported me, though they never understood why anyone would want to do such a thing (they still don't).

All the exchange students arrived on a chartered flight to Los Angeles, then boarded different connecting flights. My final destination was Virginia Beach, so I made multiple connections, each time with fewer and fewer fellow exchange students. On the final leg, I was the only one from the program, and I was seated next to a middle-aged man traveling with his two sons in their early teens.

The man was clearly curious about me and proceeded to engage me in a friendly chat. He was patient with my limited English and seemed genuinely delighted that I was spending a year in the United States. He made sure I was well taken care of for the entire flight, helping me talk to the attendants, making sure I understood the seat-belt sign and so on.

For most Americans (including me, now), this is nothing. We do these kinds of things routinely, without even thinking about it. Even sixteen-year-old me knew this was "kindness" with a lowercase "k." All the same, his open, casual friendliness—of a sort less familiar in Japan—was one of the first signs that the U.S. was indeed what I had hoped it would be, and that maybe someday, I would be welcomed to join it.

That was thirty-five years ago. After the exchange-student program, I came back to America to attend college. I've lived here ever since, and I consider it my one and only home, though I maintain Japanese citizenship, mostly to avoid further heartache for my mother. I still think of the good-hearted American on that flight so many years ago and I am grateful that his small act of kindness helped ease my transition.

You Can't Buy Class
By Kathie Klarreich

I look around: a sea of blue uniforms. There are no familiar faces in this new class of inmates. They look at me. I look back. None of us let on what we're thinking—that's a survival tactic in prison. But since this is my show, I assume an air of authority I'm not yet comfortable wearing, and I begin to talk about the content we'll cover and what I expect from them during the Exchange for Change twelve-week writing course.

Among the crop of students, two guys stand out. One resembles your average white supremacist; the other is sleeved in tattoos to his fingertips. I think there are tattoos on his eyelids. I wonder if there's a story there.

My job is to gently pick at the protective layer these men wear over their innermost thoughts and feelings. By week three, that layer has thinned. A conversation flows between these men who didn't know each other before this class. They keep coming back—except the one I'd pegged as a white supremacist.

I ask where he's gone. Locked up, they tell me.

"Locked up?" I didn't know prisoners could go to jail in prison.

They explain that he's gone to "confinement." We talk about this a little, and the following week I bring in an essay by the writer Eula Bliss to further our discussion in a tangential sort of way. The essay is about the invention of telephone poles—or at least that's what it appears to be about, until Bliss starts to list, in chronological order, how certain poles have been used for lynching.

I'm a few copies short, so I send one of my students to the office to make some more. An officer, normally friendly, smiles as she enters the classroom and leaves them on my desk. We're reading the essay aloud when this same officer returns a few minutes later and demands I hand her the copies she's just given me. She's no longer smiling. Two minutes later the director of education comes in.

"Get your stuff, and come with me," she says.

I fight to keep my face neutral of fear. Or anger. I'm a volunteer; this woman hasn't hired me. Her office is at the end of the hall, and the berating starts as soon as she shuts the classroom door behind me.

"What are you trying to do, incite a riot?" she says.

I'm not sure what she's talking about. "If you have an objection to my choice of material, I'm happy to discuss that." My speech is controlled, measured. "But I am a volunteer and a professional. I will not be humiliated. I will not be treated like an inmate."

She appears both shocked and amused. I wonder if anyone has ever stood up to her before. There's a moment of silence. Then she laughs. "Oh, you know me," she says, and suggests I teach *Harry Potter*—something fun and entertaining. Ten minutes later she's encouraging me to return to my classroom.

As I walk back down the hall, my empathy for my students grows, my respect for these men who come to class and actually find the courage to express themselves in an environment designed to silence them. When I open the door there is a collective nod.

I glance at the guy with the tattoos. I can make out the tattoo on his eyelids now. Left says "No." Right says "Evil." I pick up where I'd left off, speaking with an authority I feel I'd just earned.

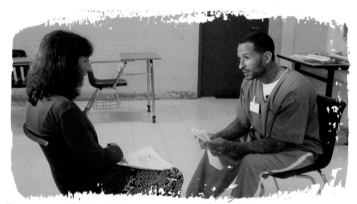

I'm nervous when I return to class the following week. The guys are already inside. We start with introductions, and then the man with the tattoos says he'd like to go first.

He starts quietly and quickly, and immediately his classmates tell him to slow down and speak up. Now I'm smiling—they sound like me. He starts again.

"You Can Pay for School but You Can't Buy Class," he begins. His story is a treatise on the way our sessions have unfolded, an appreciation of the dignity the men feel in the classroom, a railing against the kind of indignity that rains down upon them always—and had rained down on me, too, the week before.

Each week, I tell my students it's okay to be silent after someone has read in order to absorb the meaning of the piece. I fear we could be silent for days. This wildly gifted man, quiet in his struggle to preserve his pride while imprisoned, beaten by a punitive rather than rehabilitative system, has just shown through his narrative expression how to rise above it all with kindness, courage and class. In the end, he is the real teacher.

Kindness in the Workplace

Kindness is key to success in the workplace. Not only will work feel better, but productivity will be enhanced. Remember the mirror neurons I described in the introduction? They are the portion of your brain that fire in direct response to what you see and are responsible for imitation, empathy and learning. Scientists like Dr. Elaine Hatfield who study organizational behavior have demonstrated that emotions are contagious. They flow from the most powerful person in the room, and negative emotions are easier to catch than positive ones. Many of us spend more waking hours at work than at home. Rarely can we select the people we are surrounded with, and yet their emotions become our emotions via our mirror neurons. Bosses who are kind and create a positive work environment are able to drive their companies to greater heights. They can increase morale, decrease absenteeism and retain employees for longer.

Kim Cameron's doctoral work at the University of Michigan centered on the positive relationships that can emerge in organizations as a result of certain practices. Along with colleague Emma Seppela, Ph.D. at Stanford, she recommends the following to improve the workplace:

- Caring for, being interested in and maintaining responsibility for colleagues as friends.

- Providing support for one another, including offering kindness and compassion when others are struggling.

- Avoiding blame and forgiving mistakes.

- Inspiring one another at work.

- Emphasizing the meaningfulness of the work.

- Treating one another with respect, gratitude, trust and integrity.

It Gets Better
By Kathryn Arnold

It was the end of a long night, the sort that has become, in my memory, emblematic of my twenties: a night of caution, excitement, need. I was a handful of years into a dying marriage. My family lived three thousand miles away. I was lonelier than I had imagined was possible, in a city with a talent for exacerbating loneliness. I was very, very young, though it didn't feel that way.

That long night, on the humid back patio of a sweet little bar in Queens, a friend had just told me he was getting married. He had found the love of his life. He showed me the ring. He wondered aloud how he should ask. Would she say yes? Of course she would. Surely she would.

"God," he said, "it feels so good, and so crazy, to find the person you're really, totally, actually supposed to be with."

I wish I could say I made a convincing show of excitement, that I was generous enough to let him have his happiness. I wish I could say I set my own sad self aside and, in a moment of beatific grace, accepted that joy was not a zero-sum game, that my friend finding the right person didn't mean that I couldn't someday do the same. These were the things I wanted to convey. These were the things I should have conveyed. But a broken-hearted person can only do so much. And so this is what I said instead: "Congratulations on signing up for a lifetime of misery, like the rest of us."

He had the grace to laugh.

After we said goodnight, my friend mounted his bike, and I walked down the street to the 7 train, heading toward Times Square. It was two in the morning but the subway cars were half full of chattering young people, some carrying leftovers from dinner, most glassy-eyed from drink. I took a seat on the scratched plastic bench, tipsy myself, and I tried to fend off what I knew was coming: tears, warm and bitter, for the prison I had made for myself and for how gracelessly I had made my sadness another's problem. I had failed in every way I could think of: at being a friend, at being a wife, at finding the kind of unsullied love Joey had been so happy to find.

It was a full minute before I realized how intensely I was crying: streaming tears ran down each cheek, joining in a single stream beneath my chin, soaking my blouse. The 7 train was configured such that two rows of people faced each other from opposite sides of the car, and as it gently rocked its way toward Manhattan, I realized I was being observed. A row of frowning people stared at my pink face, glancing away if my eyes caught theirs.

This miserable city, I thought.

"You okay?" a voice asked. It had an Irish accent.

I turned to my left. A bearded man in a wool cap grinned at me.

"I'm fine," I said. "Sorry to make a scene."

"You want to tell me about it?"

I shook my head, my throat closing. "Just a rough night."

"I've had some of those," he said.

I smiled, not sure what to say. A beat passed.

"If I knew a joke," he said, "I'd tell it to you."

I laughed.

The train slowed, pulling into Bryant Park. The man stood, preparing to exit. As he passed in front of me to reach the door, he patted the crown of my head.

"Whatever it is, it's going to get better," he said.

There's no reason why this statement—the blandest of sympathies, the most obvious and threadbare bit of encouragement—should have moved me as it did. My only theory is that I knew, in some way opaque even to me, that he was right. I would get over this. I would be happy for my friend. I would solve my marital problems, or I would leave. If I stayed, I would find a way to be okay; if I left, I would find a way to be okay.

There were other things that would get better, though, that I couldn't have anticipated. I couldn't have guessed that one night, long after my marriage had ended, I'd go see a band and be stunned by a man's request to buy me a beer, and that this beer would turn into a seven-hour conversation, a shared home, a marriage, parenthood, the sort of love my friend had been so happy to find: the sort that makes commitment and responsibility a joy and a privilege.

Whatever it is, it will get better—this was the stranger's assurance to me, but it's also a law of nature. Things tend to improve. They evolve, strengthen, simplify. The young grow up. Broken hearts mend. That which isn't meant to be rarely lasts. And when the strange storm of youth has subsided, all that remains is what is real and true: an errant life repaired, a husband who is gloriously, thrillingly, enough.

Coincidentally, he's Irish. And he knows plenty of jokes.

"Wherever there is a human being, there is an opportunity for a kindness."
—Lucius Annaeus Seneca

Is Kindness Sexy?

Yes! Two leading evolutionary psychologists, David Buss and Michael Barnes, studied what makes people attracted to one another. Guess what topped the list? Kind and understanding took the number-one spot for both men and women. Next came exciting personality, intelligent, physically attractive, healthy, easy-going, creative, wants children, college graduate and good earning capacity. Another study, led by researchers at the University of Nottingham and Liverpool John Moores University, found that both sexes rated potential partners for a long-term relationship as more attractive when they were told the person was involved in altruistic acts such as volunteer work or caring for an older person.

So it's pretty simple: if you want to catch a great mate, Bekindr!

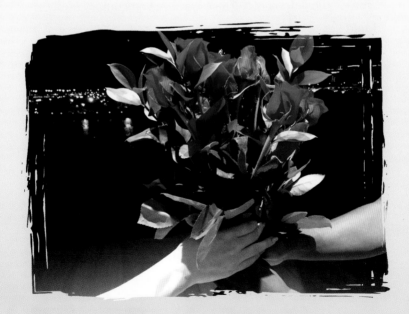

Room for Kindness
By Dhardra Blake

I was leaving an evening event and I was heading to my car when suddenly there was a huge commotion: someone smashed into a parked car. For a moment, everyone stood frozen in shock. The owner of the car was standing right there and was, understandably, quite upset. As he stood with his wife and their guest, they wondered aloud how the rest of their night would unfold: How long would it take for the police to come? Did they all need to wait? The guest was saying he had to get to work really early the next day. The wife was concerned about the children, who were waiting up for them on a school night.

"Would you like a ride?" I asked.

"Sure," the wife said. "Which way are you going?"

I told her.

"Oh," she said, then: "No thank you since that's out of your way."

"I don't mind at all," I said.

We arrived at my car. The wife and her guest popped in and we headed to her home while her husband waited to deal with the police. When we arrived, they thanked me profusely, and she and I decided to become Facebook friends.

Fast-forward three years. I posted on Facebook that I was looking for a place to stay. I had been working on yachts as a freelance chef for some months, and I was about to take a temporary land-based job. Money was tight, and it was tough to find a reasonable short-term rental. Could anyone help?

The woman I had driven home that long-ago night reached out almost immediately, even though we hadn't interacted much since our first meeting. She explained that she was going through a divorce and lived in a large home with her children. Her husband had just moved out, and it was a tough time for everyone involved. She said she would enjoy the company, and if I would cook on occasion, I could stay for free.

Gratefully I accepted her offer and moved in. I helped with the meals and getting the house in order. She provided a roof over my head, companionship and guidance as I launched my own business. We lived together for several months, and my friend's sadness over her divorce began to fade—as my new business began to grow.

When her house finally sold, we went our separate ways. But we remain the dearest of friends. That friendship started out of a small act of kindness and grew tenfold when that act was reciprocated.

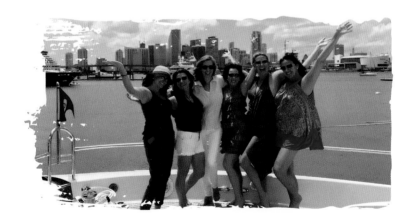

How Kindness Spreads

Researchers James H. Fowler, at the University of California, San Diego and Nicholas A. Christakis, at Harvard University explain in their compelling book, *Connected: The Surprising Power of Our Social Networks and How They Change Our Lives*, that "cooperative behavior cascades in human social networks," which is a fancy way of saying good behavior gets passed on in groups. Of course, the opposite is true as well, but that's a topic for other books. People are influenced by others' actions—typically up to three degrees of separation. If you perform a simple act of kindness, you can expect the recipient to continue this behavior and the next recipient will as well! We call this the ripple effect of kindness. Mirror neurons make us all natural imitators.

As you read earlier, Dr. Jonathan Haidt described "elevation," which comes from receiving or merely watching acts of kindness. Our bodies secrete oxytocin, and we are more likely to feel trust and warmth toward those around us and to have a genuine desire to be helpful. In technical terms, we see an increase in prosocial behavior following the release of oxytocin. In simple terms, kindness creates more kindness.

I was checking out in the market the other day, and the young man bagging my groceries offered me his coupon for a free rotisserie chicken. Yes, it was just a free chicken—but I was so surprised and touched it made my day. I had been caught in my own head, in which a long to-do list swirled. I had my nose in my phone—I hadn't even acknowledged the young man. He, on the other hand, was fully engaged in the present moment and had observed that I was spending over $40, which was the requirement for the coupon.

When he handed it to me, I felt tears well up in my eyes. I was surprised by how moved I was. I thanked him and went to my car feeling elated. This small gesture made my spirits soar.

A few minutes later, while at a red light, I saw a man on the opposite side of the street asking for money. This time, instead of staying in my own head, I waved and called him over. I excitedly handed him money just as the light was changing— so excitedly, in fact, that before I knew what I was doing, I'd blown him a kiss. He blew one back! I realized it was pretty odd behavior, but I was riding the high from the kindness I had just received, and I was just happy to be passing it on. Dr. Haidt was right. Kindness elevates us!

Pay-it-forward lines, in which someone pays for the order behind them, are an excellent demonstration of the ripple effects of kindness. The often-cited example happened at a drive-through Starbucks in St. Petersburg, Florida, at seven a.m., when a customer paid for her iced coffee and then paid for the caramel macchiato ordered by the customer behind her. The barista continued to explain the process to each subsequent customer, and the process continued for an astounding 378 people. Everyone accepted a free drink and paid for the customer behind them, all the way up until six p.m., when the 379th person ordered a coffee and declined to pay for the next one. The barista felt the chain had been broken simply because that customer didn't understand the concept.

Another interesting part of the story that hasn't been reported is what happened to the 378 people who received kindness that day. Research suggests that, in addition to being kind to the person behind them, they were most likely elevated by the experience and showed kindness to two others. Let's do the math: 378 x 2 more people each equals 756. Then 756 x 3 = 2,268 and then one more round 2,268 x 3 = 6,804. Add all those together, and you get 10,206. So it's possible that the one cup of coffee generated over 10,000 other acts of kindness. Not bad for a $5 investment.

When collecting stories for Bekindr, there was often a discrepancy between how the giver and the receiver felt about the exchange. The giver often felt that he or she had not done all that much. That's probably the way the first person in the Starbucks line felt at seven that morning. They were simply doing what they thought anyone would do. The receiver, on the other hand, often felt profoundly moved by the experience and was very grateful, reminding us that "a little often goes a long way." One small cup of coffee, bought for the right person at the right time, can indeed set off a chain reaction, one that begins to change the world for the better.

Another beautiful example of the ripple effects of kindness occurred in February 2014, when an eight-year-old boy named Myles Ecker found a $20 bill in the parking lot of a Cracker Barrel in Toledo, Ohio. He said, "I kind of wanted to get a video game but then I decided not to." He changed his mind when he saw a guy in a uniform who reminded him of his dad. Myles's dad had been killed in Iraq just five weeks after Myles was born. Myles handed the soldier a sticky note with the following message:

"Dear Soldier—my dad was a soldier. He's in heaven now. I found this 20 dollars in the parking lot when we got here. We like to pay it forward in my family. It's your lucky day! Thank you for your service."

Myles Eckert, a Gold Star Kid*

This simple act of kindness created many ripples. The story went viral and was seen on TV and social media. Myles was invited to appear on *Ellen* and visit with President George W. Bush at his presidential library. He received the Medal

*Gold Star Children was founded in 2008 to raise awareness about American children who lost a parent while serving in the U.S. military.

of Honor to recognize citizens who have gone above their call of duty. Myles's family is now spearheading a nonprofit organization called the "Power of 20" with the goal of giving on an even greater scale to charities and families in need. Recently, they provided a dying soldier his final wish of attending a Green Bay Packers playoff game. Myles remained by his side and provided comfort to the soldier on his final day. He then served as an honorary pallbearer at the soldier's funeral.

Good thing Myles didn't buy that video game!

"Kindness gives birth to kindness."
—*Sophocles*

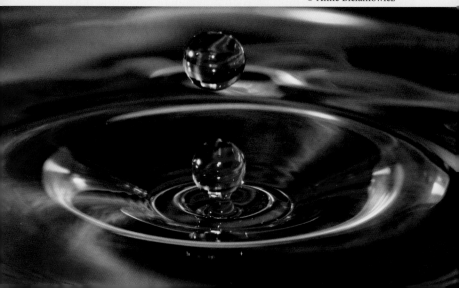

This Little Light
By Jen Waldron

"I think you should come," my dad said through the phone.

"Is everything alright?" I asked. "I just talked to the nurse last night, and she said Mom was doing a bit better."

"Yeah," he said. "I asked her if she wanted you kids to be here, and she nodded."

My mom was lying in a hospital bed in Maine, far from my Georgia home. As I headed north with my sister, I knew. My dad would never ask us to be there unless it was necessary. My mother was going to die.

I sat by her bedside as she slept, under sedation. Machines allowed her to breathe. The doctor met with us as a family. "There is nothing more I can do," he said. But that wasn't entirely true. Because what he did do was sit and talk with us for a long time, sharing stories of my mother, telling us how much he loved her sense of humor.

"Your wife, your mother, is an amazing person," the doctor said. "I have enjoyed getting to know her. She always has a smile on her face, and when she visits, I end up smiling, too."

I liked knowing that he had seen her, not just her illness.

The machines soon fell silent, and it was time to say goodbye. As we entered the room, numb and sad, the staff asked for a moment more to ready our mother. I stood outside the curtain and watched them give her the gentlest treatment.

They washed her from head to toe, soothed her skin with lotion, moistened her dry lips and styled her hair. She was treated as though she were getting ready to go somewhere special. I suppose she was.

When the curtain parted, we gathered at her side. My mother looked peaceful. The room was quiet, tidy. I noticed her feet. The nurses had found the funny little socks I'd bought for my mother at a nearby store. I knew she would smile at them if she could. Swallowing a lump in my throat, I gave thanks for this deed, this small gesture of kindness.

It is sad to say goodbye, of course. When she left this earth, we grieved. For my dad, her husband of more than fifty years, it was too much. My sister and I tried to ask about arrangements, and he said he couldn't do it. We asked if we should and he said yes.

The sky outside was gray and cold; snow flurries blew all around. My sister and I headed back to the hotel to begin handling what needed to be done. The hotel staff was helpful and patient as we tied up their fax machines and office area with reams of unhappy documents. It was hard, but we tried to be as brave and wise as Mom had been.

Eventually, we took a break for dinner at a local chowder house by the sea that Mom had loved. Seagulls flew across the winter sky. We shared memories and laughter through our tears and ordered bowls of the lobster bisque our mother had especially enjoyed.

When we returned to the hotel and opened the door to our room, there was a card on the floor. Inside was a note from the hotel staff:

> *Nothing can make this day better.*
> *Please accept this stay on us.*
> *It is the least we can do.*

The kindnesses of that day remain with me still. The genuine words from a doctor I'd just met. The socks on my mother's feet—such a small but essential act—for her journey to the other side. The generosity of the hotel and their handwritten note. Each act lifted the darkness of sorrow and allowed light to shine in.

Thunder
By Jessica Kizorek

I am a media producer who specializes in fundraising videos for philanthropic organizations. For one particularly far-flung assignment, I traveled to Burkina Faso, West Africa. I had been hired by an organization called Women Thrive to show how the organization influenced legislation in Washington, D.C. to ensure foreign aid was allocated to women and girls around the world.

So there I was, in this tiny landlocked African country, looking out the window onto a landscape straight out of *National Geographic.* To paint a picture for you, this is the kind of place where the village chief gives you a live goat and rooster after introducing you to his thirteen wives and fifty-six children. In that part of the world, animals are extremely valuable, so a gift of that nature was an ultimate act of kindness. I was moved by this generosity—even though we had to strap the goat to the roof rack for a three-hour road trip back to the city.

Animals ended up being a big theme of the trip. The day after we received the goat and chicken, we interviewed the head of the women's farming cooperative, Maryam. I asked her what she needed most. She said they really needed a farm animal to help them plow the modest plot of land on which they grew vegetables.

In Burkina Faso, men own 99 percent of the land and animals. So this livestock donation—given directly to the women of the village—would be a major breakthrough, not only for their vegetable yield but also for their self-sufficiency and for extras their subsistence-level farming could not support. The money the women made as a collective was important; their disposable income from vegetable sales meant they could pool funds for expenses we take for granted, like emergency medical care or the ability to send the most promising kids in the village to school. On rare occasions, they purchased salt or spices for special celebratory meals—a luxury their husbands could rarely afford.

Maryam told me that day, in no uncertain terms, that a donkey or a cow was at the top of their list. I felt a certain burden of responsibility to make it happen for them. They were going to get this farm animal if it was the last thing I did.

The first problem I faced was that I had no idea how much these animals cost. I had never purchased a live donkey or cow. Plus, it had to be an awesome, productive one. Not sickly, like many of the animals I saw in Burkina. After a little digging, I found that a donkey cost around $225.

Later that night, I was about to head to bed when I opened up my backpack and found the small sum of cash I'd set aside for souvenirs. Africa has the most amazing shopping—the best handicrafts in the world, carved wooden masks I loved to bring home to friends. But now I felt torn.

I counted the stack. It came to $241. I was convinced this was no accident. I could buy ten masks for friends. Or I could buy a single donkey, skipping a stone into the world of these women, with ripple effects that would reach their children and their children's children. The more I thought about this, the more clearly I understood what I needed to do.

A few more days passed before I prepared for the trek back to the airport. It was time to leave. Over coffee on my last morning in Burkina, I sat down with the liaison and translator, who had been by my side the entire trip. I pulled out a thick envelope from my carry-on. I explained that the money came with three conditions: First, the donkey it purchased had to be handsome, healthy and strong. Second, they had to name it *Tonnerre*—thunder, in their native French. Finally, they had to take a picture of themselves with this glorious beast and send it to me.

On the one hand, it felt like a big deal. On the other, it felt so small. Here I was, filming a video to help lawmakers decide how billions in United States foreign aid would be divided. Two hundred and twenty-five dollars wasn't going to build a hospital or fund a school. But then I realized that, while sometimes kindness is a profound and expensive gesture, often it's the smallest acts that make a difference.

I hadn't expected how much the photo would impact me when it arrived almost six months later. But when it popped up on my computer one afternoon, I knew it was a day I'd never forget.

I'll never know the true impact of *Tonnerre* in that community. But I do know how grateful I was I had an opportunity to try to make a difference. Sometimes it takes an experience on the other side of the world to realize that no matter what's exchanged, the universal laws of kindness are always the same: It feels good to give. It feels good to receive. And, it always feels good to remember it.

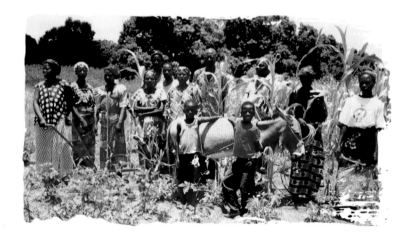

A Cup of Kindness
By Joy Marinoff

It was a frigid December afternoon in Pennsylvania, and I stood on the street, covered in layers, shivering bitterly. I wore gloves, but they did little to warm my hands, and as I held out a bucket to passing cars, soliciting donations for pediatric cancer research, I jumped around to try to keep warm. My friends—native Philadelphians—often joked that I, a Floridian, couldn't take the weather. They were right. Hours into our outdoor adventure, I'd only received a few dollars.

Then two things happened that changed the day entirely.

First, a car drove by and the driver hid a hundred-dollar bill in a one-dollar bill, dropping it in and speeding away without a word. It was hours before we realized what they had done.

Not long after, an older gentleman got out of his car and handed me some change. I thanked him for his donation. Thirty minutes later, he returned. He handed me a cup of hot chocolate. "You looked cold," he said, "and I appreciate what you're doing out here." He smiled, his rosy cheeks beaming.

He didn't know me. In fact, he knew nothing about me. All he knew was that I was cold, and that was enough for him to carry out an act that warmed my heart more than any cup of hot chocolate could.

> "If you want more kindness in the world, put some there."
>
> —Zera Dean

Can Kindness Cure Disease?

O ne of the best example of kindness curing disease can be found in Alcoholics Anonymous (AA), where groups of strangers come together with the sole purpose of aiding one another and thereby aiding themselves, to battle a potentially lethal disease.

In 1934, Bill Wilson got sober with a lot of help. It took the aid of hospitalization, the encouragement of a friend who had made his own dramatic recovery, a spiritual awakening and the care of a wise and compassionate physician who saw alcoholism as a disease rather than a character flaw. Folklore has it that after Bill left the hospital, he wandered around the streets and talked to "drunks" about the importance of getting sober. After several months and no luck, he came home and complained to his wife that he has been tirelessly trying to treat alcoholics, and none were getting sober. She cleverly quipped back, "But you are." So Bill continued to try to aid others.

Shortly thereafter, while on a business trip to Akron, Ohio, he felt a strong urge to drink. In his hotel lobby, he looked at the directory of churches and selected one at random. He made a call and asked the minister, "Is there a hopeless drunk I can talk to?" His next call was to a surgeon named Robert Smith, and they spoke for hours. Bill's urge to drink passed. Dr. Bob, as he has come to be known, also never took another drink, and together they co-founded AA based on the notion that helping others was a key element to obtaining and maintaining their own sobriety. Approximately 2 million people belong to AA and attend over 100,000 meeting groups in 181 countries. Bill W. has been recognized as one of the "greatest social architects" and listed in *Time Magazine*'s "100 Heroes and Icons of the Twentieth Century" for his simple concept of treating his disease by caring for strangers.

HALTing My Disease
By Anonymous

Nothing was wrong with me…or so I thought. I was forty-four years old, on top of my game in the accounting firm where I work and making lots of money. My wife could be a bit of a nag, but lots of my friends felt the same way about their wives, and the kids were doing great. So when I went to my internist for my annual checkup, I was quite surprised when he told me to stop drinking.

"Why?" I asked. I thought he was nuts. So I had a few scotches after work? And what was the big deal about going out with friends on the weekend?

The internist mumbled something about my liver enzymes but I paid no attention. He was just overreacting.

Christmas came, and our family went on a ski trip. While we were skiing, my stomach began to hurt. It's nothing, I told myself. I spent a day in bed, and it passed.

On April 16th, having survived another tax season, I decided to celebrate. I went out to dinner with the firm's partners and had a few drinks. I didn't feel so good afterward, so I went home and tried to sleep. The pain got worse. I woke my wife, and she said we needed to go to the emergency room. The pain was intense by that time, so I agreed.

"You have pancreatitis," the doctor said.

What?

He told me I needed to stay in the hospital for a bit and as long as I didn't drink, I'd be fine.

A few days passed uneventfully, and I was ready to go home.

No drinking? Well, I could do that…or so I thought. The first week wasn't hard. I was regaining my strength, and my stomach pain was diminishing. I was enjoying the time with my wife and kids. My wife said I seemed different, but I wasn't really sure what she meant.

Two weeks passed, and we were invited to a friend's fiftieth birthday party. It was great. Amazing food and wine. Without even thinking about it, I had a glass. The pain returned. This is ridiculous, I thought to myself. Must be something I ate, but just in case, I put the glass down.

Another three weeks passed, and I was still staying away from alcohol. Maybe this won't be so bad. I had more energy in the morning, was hitting the gym early and had been more focused at work. My wife continued to say she liked the new me.

One Friday, the guys were going for a happy hour. My wife and kids were at my son's basketball game, so I joined them, knowing my family wouldn't be home for a few hours. What happened next is not clear. All I know is that I ended up back in the emergency room. Different doctor, more pain, and this time, I'd hit my head. The doctor did a CT scan and said I was a lucky guy. I didn't even know what he was talking about. "Better lay off the sauce," he said and patted me on the back. What was happening? What should I tell my wife? He told me to see my own doctor on Monday. I sheepishly headed home and crawled into bed. My wife looked panicked when she saw me. I told her I needed to rest.

The next day I told her I couldn't remember anything that had happened except that I'd left the office to meet the guys and woke up in the E.R. She wanted to call the guys but I begged her not to. The confusion, fear and anger I saw in her face rattled me to my core. Maybe she was right. Maybe the doctor was right. This time I resolved to do something about my drinking.

On Monday, my wife and I went together to my internist. He said my pancreas was fine and told me he thought I'd had an alcoholic blackout. He went on to say that alcohol is actually a poison, and our liver needs to detoxify it and mine wasn't able to. Kids in college, whose livers aren't accustomed to drinking, more frequently get alcohol poisoning. Some even die.

He said I'd never had a blackout before because I was a regular drinker. That was true. Now that I hadn't been drinking for several weeks, I was at greater risk. The amount I had consumed with the guys that night was too much for my system.

"So what do I do?" I asked him.

He said I had a few choices. One was checking myself into a rehabilitation facility, where I would be unable to get alcohol and could give my brain a chance to heal and learn about the disease and new ways to cope. It usually takes a month. It might be covered by insurance, depending on where I went. That sounded challenging. How could I ever explain that to my boss and kids?

"What other options are there?" I asked.

"Well," he said, "You could try Alcoholics Anonymous. It's free, and there are meetings everywhere, many times a day."

That sounded much easier, so I agreed.

Walking into my first meeting was overwhelming. It was filled with about twenty-five men and women, all of whom sat in a circle and took turns telling their stories. They each said they were an alcoholic and were powerless over alcohol. They had stories far worse than mine. Maybe I was right, and I didn't really need to be here. But then I remembered the look on my wife's face and I stayed.

After the meeting, a man approached me and introduced himself as Tony. He said he had been sober for twenty years and he would like to be my sponsor. "What's that?" I asked. He explained that AA follows many simple steps, and one was to get a sponsor. Someone you could talk to anytime. Someone to help you and guide you to a new life of sobriety. The sponsor is a combination of a coach, a friend and a therapist. They take you through the twelve steps of recovery. Tony looked like a good guy, so I shook his hand, and the rest, as they say, is history.

From Tony and the AA meetings, I learned ways to avoid drinking. He taught me to look for triggers when I have an urge to drink and taught me the acronym HALT: Hungry, Angry, Lonely, Tired. He attended happy hours with me and the guys the first few times and taught me to order a soda or fruit drink as soon as I arrived and keep it in my hand so no one offered me anything else. We began playing tennis together and he helped me shift my schedule so I looked forward to getting up early and avoided late dinners and parties with a lot of drinking. He guided me to give up friends who, I now realized, were drinking too much. I made new friends in AA. Tony and I talked every day.

Tony never got paid for all the time he invested in me and my recovery. He explained that this was how AA worked. All members and sponsors are volunteers there to help themselves and help one another. I feel I owe my health and happiness to Tony and all the others at AA. Five years have passed, and now I am a sponsor of someone at AA. He reminds me of my former self, and it helps me see how far I have come. I continue to attend meetings three times a week. Tony and I talk at the meetings and outside of them, as well. I have learned to be a better husband, father and accountant and I have come to appreciate that although I can never be cured of alcoholism, every day I don't drink, I am successfully battling the disease. AA is free and has meetings just about everywhere, including online. Join us if you need help. We are here for you!

> "The best portion of a good man's life: his little nameless, unremembered acts of kindness and love."
> —William Wordsworth

Stranded in the Chill
By Craig Calvert

My wife, young son, and I lived in a remote area of the Ozarks. When the first winter came, I was woefully unprepared and inexperienced—I had come from Baltimore where I'd zipped around in a small hatchback. That hatchback was just as woefully unprepared as I was for life on the side of a rocky mountain.

Two weeks after we moved to our mountain home, I got caught in the beginnings of a snowstorm while coming back from the nearest grocery store which was ten miles away. As I drove up the mountain, the snow started coming down hard. Then, about a mile from home, my car stopped going up and instead, began to slide backward...for the longest fifteen seconds of my life. Luckily, it stopped before reaching the steep embankment.

So there I was, wearing only a hoodie and without gloves, stranded in the chill. I started to walk the rest of the way. Within minutes, a local drove by in a big four-wheel-drive truck. He stopped, made a few cackling remarks about my diminutive car and hooked a big chain to its fender. He never asked how far away my home was. He didn't even ask if I needed help. He simply dove in and did what needed to be done, and I am certain he wouldn't have blinked if I had said my home was twenty miles away.

Once I was seated in his truck (the heat felt so good—I was so cold I could barely move my lips), he asked where we were headed.

"Just about a mile, right where the truck rig is parked."

His eyes lit up. "You live near the Applings! They're good people."

I had to admit that I had just recently moved to the area and had not yet met the Applings. To be fair, "neighbor" is a rather relative term in the Ozarks. "Next door" could mean several miles, and as it turned out, the Applings lived some distance up the road.

A few minutes later, we arrived at the dirt road on which I lived, got my car parked safely off the main highway, and we shook hands. "Tell Joe that Billy says hi!" the man said, and then he was back on the highway.

It was two weeks before the highway became passable again, and I decided to try to get my car from the highway back up to my house. What I didn't factor in was that the highway had been salted, but my dirt road had definitely not been. The road was heavily shaded by trees and still had lots of ice hanging around. About halfway up, my car slid into a ditch. I was, for the second time in as many weeks, totally stuck.

Like magic, the fabled Joe Appling appeared with two cans of Bud Light. "You must be the new folks! Looks like you took an unexpected detour." He handed me a beer. "I'll be right back."

A few minutes later, I heard a tractor rumbling toward me. Joe inched up carefully to the car, and like a master craftsman, delicately (and rapidly) maneuvered the backhoe under my car. Deftly, he brought it back out of the ditch—one-handed, while holding his beer.

Over the next few months, I got to know the Applings well. Joe often gave me mountain-living tips (always shared over just slightly cool cans of Bud Light), and we often crossed paths on our single dirt road and chatted. Over time, I began to feel as though I could make it out there on the mountain—and that was thanks, in large part, to the kindness I was shown in that new and foreign place.

The next year, just before winter rolled around, I cut down some trees that had been damaged by the previous year's ice storm. I processed three large trees for firewood and was feeling really good about myself. Unfortunately, unbeknownst to me, the three trees I had cut down were all white oak. White oak, it turns out, is among the worst choices for firewood. You could douse a pile of white oak with gasoline, and it still might not burn. So, one day I got on Facebook and griped about having all this firewood I couldn't use. I spent days taking the white oak out of my wood stack, grumbling the entire time.

Not long after, I received some sad news: Joe Appling had died. He had gone out hunting and killed a deer, and when he tried to take it back up the mountain, his ATV flipped over and crushed him.

Two days later, I saw Terry, his wife, walking down the road, crying. When she got close, I could tell she had been crying for a long time. She turned to me and said, "Can you help me?"

"Anything, Terry!" I said.

"Could you come get all the firewood at my place? The last thing Joe did before he left for the last time was chop wood. I can't look at that pile anymore. I want you to have it."

I had always heard the adage, "I cried because I had no shoes until I met a man who had no feet." In this moment, Terry taught me what this really meant.

Joe's generosity has always stuck with me. Even after his death, he managed to help out someone he cared about—someone who, I think he realized, needed all the help he could get.

"Human kindness has never weakened the stamina or softened the fiber of free people. A nation does not have to be cruel to be tough."

—Franklin Delano Roosevelt

Wildfire
By Praveen Yalamanchi

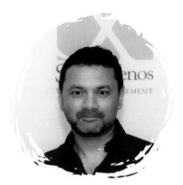

My dad had purchased a Jeep Wrangler for me for my sixteenth birthday (in fact, he got it while I was still fifteen so I could start learning with my learner's permit). It was stick shift—he wanted to force me to learn stick, feeling that otherwise, I'd go a lifetime without attempting to learn it.

After several weekends of learning to drive the new car with my dad, I felt comfortable enough to go out on my own. The first trip was driving my younger brothers to the toy store to buy a new video-game system. I still have the canceled check from Toys"R"Us. This was before the era of teens having their own credit cards, but parents commonly opened savings accounts with limited check-writing privileges to teach their kids money management.

In Florida, like the rest of the country, we have four seasons, but in our state, they're hurricane season, fire season, wet season and dry season. Fire season is around springtime after the long, dry winter months have parched the Florida Everglades, and there's a spike in dry-weather lightning strikes on the dry grassy swamplands.

Our neighborhood is not far from the Everglades. One weekend, we woke up with a lot of smoke in the air. Turning on the TV news, we saw brush fires in the Everglades. Being genius sixteen-year-olds, hungry for life and adventure, my best friend, who lived across the street from me, his step-brother, and I took off the top of my Jeep Wrangler and set off to find the wildfires. I was motivated by the romance of off-roading that I'd seen in Jeep marketing campaigns and in movies.

This was before cell phones and GPS, so we just set off blindly, trying to follow where the smoke was coming from. We wound up finding a hidden turn off a small highway where other off-road vehicles seemed to be congregating. It was the boundary between the highway and the edge of the Everglades, with smoke still streaming in from somewhere in the distance.

As we turned off the highway, I saw what looked like an off-roading course, complete with dirt-hill jumps over mud puddles. Years later, I would realize these were just remnants from the construction of the highway a few years before. We took the track without knowing where it led, hoping it veered close to the fire at some point, and not realizing the actual complexities or logistics of off-roading in a swamp like the Everglades with what was essentially a road vehicle.

It was such a blast hopping over mud puddles and veering between the dirt mounds! I enjoyed trying out the various four-wheel-drive settings. I soon realized that it was more fun to drive through the puddles than drive around them since the mud would splash over the front seat of the car and hit the back seat occupants. We had the top down, and the windshield protected me, while my friends were getting covered in mud.

A few minutes later, we passed a Florida highway patrol trooper in his car on the course. I don't know why he was there, but he got out of his car, came over and talked to us, asking what we were doing out here. I told him were looking for the fires. Back when I was in high school, South Florida was more rural and outdoor-friendly, so the answer didn't really faze or surprise him. He just said it was too dangerous and that we should go back.

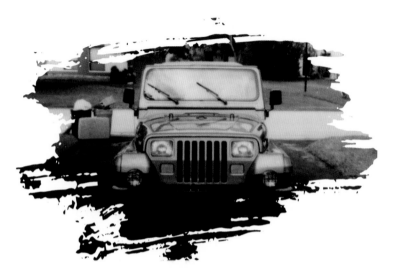

We turned around. But, not wanting to feel the day was a total loss, I sought out every mud pit as we drove, each one more fun than the last. Until…

One last pit. It seemed kind of different from the previous ones. It was shallow but very long. When we were halfway through, I could feel the engine sputter and knew it was going to stall. So I downshifted to first gear, but it didn't help. More sputtering. Finally, I made a fatal error. I stopped on purpose to shift from four-wheel-drive high to four-wheel-drive low mode, eliminating all forward momentum through the long mud pit. Once stopped, the engine sputtered to a halt. I tried cranking the engine again and again, but it wouldn't catch. We also noticed that we were slowly sinking! This was some sort of quicksand, and we were stuck. The tailpipe was under thick mud, so there was no way for the engine to restart.

I helped my friends jump to the dry spot of land parallel to the mud pit and then jumped myself after they were safe. Once the three of us were off, the Jeep stopped sinking so fast, because there was less weight on board.

Now what? We were stranded in the middle of an alligator-infested swamp, with a raging wildfire nearby.

Before we could panic, an older gentleman drove by. He was in a Ford Bronco and had a winch on the front of his truck. He was able to winch my Jeep out of the pit onto dry land. I tried starting the Jeep and it started, but it wouldn't stay running. Mud had seeped into the engine bay, contaminating the vacuum seal, so the engine would no longer automatically idle. The kind stranger gave me an impromptu driving lesson on how to drive with one foot on the brake and one the gas like they do in England. The practical effect was to always keep the foot on the gas so the engine wouldn't stall from lack of idle, but to shift into neutral when I had to slow down and brake.

I offered the kind stranger $50, which was a fortune at the time for a tenth grader. He declined and told me to do the same for someone else someday. I never saw that guy again, but his lesson ignited a chain reaction in me, and I've been fortunate enough to help many people in my lifetime of travels in the Americas and Asia. Every time someone offers thanks for an unprovoked help or major act of kindness, I always repeat what that stranger said to me and taught me that fateful day.

"May I never be too busy in my own affairs to respond to the needs of others with kindness and compassion."

—Thomas Jefferson

The Nobel Prize

Do you know the origin of the Nobel Prize? I didn't until I started researching for this book. According to Olov Amelin, curator of the Nobel Museum, the prize had a very unusual inspiration.

In 1888, Ludwig Nobel died. The French press confused him with his younger brother, Alfred, the famed Swedish inventor of dynamite and other explosive material. They ran a very negative story calling him the "Tradesman of Death," saying he was the man who made it possible to kill more people quickly than anyone who had ever lived.

Finding himself in the unusual position of reading his own obituary, Alfred was deeply saddened by this perception and he set about to ensure that his legacy would create a positive and lasting contribution to humanity.

He thought for seven years and finally devised a plan, and then he redrafted his last will and testament. He detailed the money he wanted to leave his relatives (he had no children) and staff and left the remainder (94 percent, equivalent to around two hundred million dollars today) in a fund, "The interest on which shall be annually distributed in the form of prizes to those who, during the preceding year, shall have conferred the greatest benefit to mankind."

Brilliant!

He went on to specify "One part to the person who shall have done the most or the best work for fraternity between nations, for the abolition or reduction of standing armies and for the holding and promotion of peace congress." Hence, the Nobel Peace Prize was created.

That is perhaps the best example I have ever seen of making lemonade out of lemons.

How do you want to be remembered? Many of us want to be remembered for the kind acts we have done, and it's never too early to start ensuring that legacy.

Despite the Rain
By Susan Fleming

It was 2:30 p.m. on a weekday, and I was driving home from a meeting at a local medical center. The road was used by many drivers as a throughway; my mother had driven that road by herself a number of times, going to and from the medical center. The surrounding neighborhood could be described as sketchy, at best.

Before I left the medical facility, while in the parking garage, I had an uneasy feeling, and instead of keeping my purse on the passenger seat, I moved it to the floor on the passenger side. I had almost reached the end of the throughway when the light turned red. There were cars in the lane to my right and cars in front of and behind me. I didn't have the radio on or any other distraction, and I was facing forward. Suddenly, out of nowhere, I saw a young man in my passenger window with his T-shirt pulled up to cover the bottom of his face. In less than three seconds, he broke the passenger window using some kind of device and was halfway inside my car. I honked my horn and turned toward the lane on my left but there were cars in that lane going in the other direction. I was trapped.

The young man grabbed my purse and ran off. Needless to say, I was very scared. No one stopped to help, not even the witnesses at the bus stop. One man said, "Would you look at that—he just grabbed her purse!"

I pulled over to the side of the road. A man who had seen everything from across the street came over to me. He didn't look like the most reputable person, but I was grateful for the help. I was shaking so much that I couldn't dial my cell phone to call the police. This total stranger wrapped a very traumatic experience in a big blanket of warmth and kindness and totally changed the way I recall this upsetting event. He dialed and waited with me. First, a police officer came, and my Good Samaritan described what he witnessed and provided his identifying information to the police. He continued to stay with me while I waited for the detective to arrive, despite the rain…

"It is the characteristic of the magnanimous man to ask no favor but to be ready to do kindness to others."

—Aristotle

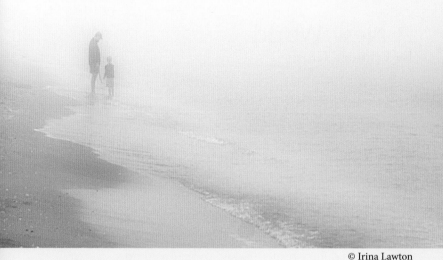

© Irina Lawton

EMPATHY

Empathy is the root of kindness and compassion. Empathy is the capacity to understand or feel what another person is experiencing from within the other person's frame of reference. "Empathy," according to physician and psychotherapist Dr. Alfred Adler, "is seeing with the eyes of another, listening with the ears of another and feeling with the heart of another." When we witness someone struggle, we can tap into our own emotions and decide how we would want to be treated, and then act accordingly.

Empathy requires effort, and we are always going to be able to be more empathic when we are in a good place ourselves. If we are rested, well fed and feeling confident and happy, it's easy to take the time to reflect on how someone else is feeling. When we are weak, tired, rushed or upset, it is difficult to find the necessary energy to give, especially to strangers. Thus, if you truly want to be a kind person, you must start with yourself. Then as you treat yourself well, so too can you do unto others.

A New World
By Frances Ghitis

Thirty years ago, my husband, Arnoldo, and I were living in Colombia with our three-year-old son and a baby on the way. Arnoldo had just finished his training as a physician and hoped to continue his specialized training in the United States. We wrote 150 letters trying to get him into a program. Though I experienced complications with my pregnancy, I did my best to help him. Finally, all the letters were typed and mailed.

He received forty responses and they all said no.

He was open to so many possibilities, but all doors seemed to be closed. He wanted to further his education and help create a better life for me and our children, and he was being denied the chance.

We started contacting everyone we could think of to ask for help. Through a series of phone calls, we reached two men, Didier and Marcos, complete strangers to my husband, who knew of hospitals that took foreign doctors for training. They each pulled as many strings as they could. Soon my husband landed an interview at Saint Luke's Hospital and was accepted for training. They became our angels.

I was still in Colombia with our two children. I had just given birth to our daughter and couldn't fly for two months. When I finally arrived, I also received such kindness from those two doctors. The night before the new medical interns started their training, there was a party and wives were expected to attend. I didn't have a babysitter. Marcos, our new friend, found the daughter of a doctor who was willing to sit for our children. Soon after, he took my husband shopping and guided us to the right area that we should find a rental house and suggested we become members of the Jewish Community Center where our son could go to camp and, later on, preschool.

Both of them looked after us, guided us through processes we barely understood. Didier and his wife (also a physician) took my husband in their home as soon as he got into Saint Luke's. In his very little free time, Didier took Arnoldo to buy a washer and dryer. He explained that we needed to buy it from Sears because we could get a credit card there, which at that time was the only credit we could get in this country. He also showed him a car dealer so he could get around on his own. He even gave us directions to every place from supermarkets to shopping malls and inexpensive furniture stores. They both told me of places to take the children for free and quality entertainment.

Soon, Marcos explained that my husband needed to move to another hospital to broaden his training—if he wanted to advance in his career, he needed to get as much experience as possible. Marcos arranged an interview for my husband with a more prestigious hospital where he was invited to transfer and train.

At this new hospital, the competition was tough. The supervising doctors were demanding, and my husband was the only foreign trainee. They didn't understand his accent. People made fun of him. He felt like a fish out of water, like he couldn't measure up. But our dear friend Marcos (who also was a foreigner and had a Spanish accent) always told my husband to keep going and not give up. He survived those difficult three years, then applied to specialize in cardiology at another prestigious hospital. He got in.

When my husband was about to finish his last year of training, he was invited to stay with the practice. We decided we wanted to live in Florida, to have more of our culture around us, and to be closer to our family in South America. Because of his great credentials and recommendations, my husband was offered a few promising possibilities, and he chose the practice in South Florida where he has been for 25 years.

He has saved so many lives and loves what he does every day. And none of that would have been possible without the strangers who became our angels, providing unconditional help above and beyond anyone's expectations, without asking anything of us in return.

"Always try to be a little kinder than is necessary."

—J.M. Barrie,
Creator of Peter Pan

Ten Pages
By Tammi Leader Fuller

My daughter was born on September 17, 1988. Shortly after her birth, I found out that she had a hole in her heart. I had an emotional breakdown. I was in the hospital, and they sent in a social worker to see me because I was such a wreck. I don't remember her name or even what she looked like. We didn't know if my baby was going to live or die. She told me that I should start writing a journal to my daughter as if she were twenty-one years old. The social worker thought I wasn't going to have my daughter around for very long and she thought I should write these letters so I could remember the brief time we would have together.

I was a journalist, and I did a lot of flying for my job. Every time my child did something cute, I would write it down on a sticky note and place it into a composition book. Then, when I got on the plane, I would weave it into a story. I wrote by hand because the social worker had told me I couldn't type the journal. Over the years, I wrote to both of my daughters as if they were grownups and told them about our life and what was happening. My husband was dealing with depression, and our marriage fell apart.

I ended up writing sixteen books for my daughters. My daughters knew about them, and they would often ask if they were old enough to read them. The only one I typed was the day I got divorced. I wrote ten pages that one day so they would really understand the circumstances. Those ten pages were tucked into the other pages of the journals.

When I moved to California in 2009, my oldest daughter was twenty-one, so I decided it was time to share the journals. We took a trip up the coast, and every day we would read one. It was shocking for them and shocking for me because so many things had been forgotten over the years. Both of my kids were blown away. My little one said, "I can't wait until my kids grow up, and you can do this for them, too."

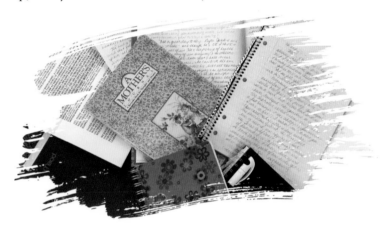

Thankfully, my daughter is now totally healthy, and as a bonus, we have these amazing archives! I have passed this idea on to numerous friends, who have created their own family journal for their daughters and sons. All because a kind woman, who knew I was facing a terrible possibility, took the time to help me channel my feelings into something positive and lasting, something that ended up becoming a cherished gift for my beloved daughter and my family.

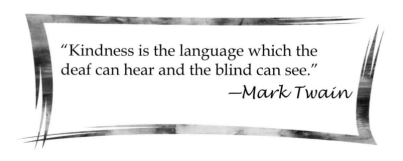

"Kindness is the language which the deaf can hear and the blind can see."

—Mark Twain

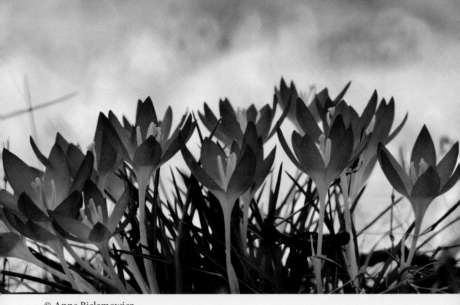

© Anne Bielamowicz

Random Acts of Flowers

Friedrich Nietzsche, a German philosopher who lived in the 1800's, said: "That which does not kill us, makes us stronger." Although I like to think the path to strength can be so much more positive, it certainly applies at times. Take, for example, Larsen Jay, who in 2007, fell off a ladder while doing some work on his roof and had to spend three weeks in the hospital convalescing. He received more than 50 floral bouquets and plants to cheer him up. Towards the end of his hospitalization, he decided to bring them to other patients whose rooms looked barren.

The joy that this act gave Jay stuck with him after he left the hospital. In 2009, he went on to create a nonprofit called Random Acts of Flowers. They now have five offices in different cities in the U.S. After an event is over, volunteers gather up flowers from weddings, memorial services, florists, special events, grocery stores, museums and churches. They reassemble the blooms into bouquets and deliver them to patients in area hospitals, assisted living facilities, hospice care centers and nursing homes. Since its inception, over 100,000 volunteer hours have been logged, and over 200,000 recipients nationwide have received flowers.

Flowers have tremendous power to lift our mood. In fact, nature often lifts our mood as we were designed to live in a much closer relationship with our environment. Flowers are a way of bringing a bit of the outside inside and can make our spirits soar. Yellow flowers often represent friendship; red roses often represent love and romance. Cherry blossoms are associated with beauty and the ethereal nature of life and kindness. Anyone who has ever been fortunate enough to visit the Tidal Basin in Washington, D.C. during the brief cherry blossom season, knows that they are a gift that keeps on giving. In 1912, Mayor Yukio Ozaki of Tokyo City gave 3,000 cherry trees to the city of Washington, D.C. as a symbol of the two countries growing friendship. Over 100 years later, they continue to delight visitors who come from around the world to view them.

© Anne Bielamowicz

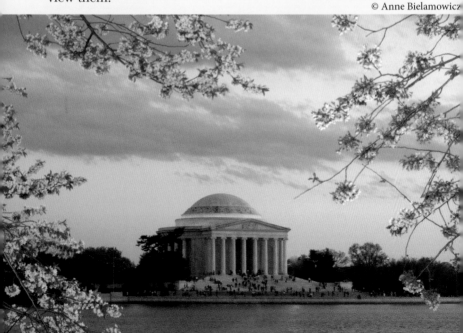

Journey of Trust
By Kerry Gruson

Competing at the Florida Ironman, Cristina Ramirez was impressed and moved by a blind competitor and her guide who together covered the 140.6-mile course, swimming, biking and running. Returning to Miami, Cristina vowed to do the same and bring the thrill of an endurance race to someone unable to do it on his or her own.

Cristina was then a forty-one-year-old triathlete, a community activist and mother. I was sixty-six, a severely disabled racing sailor and scuba diver, who refused to be defined by my disability or deterred from living at full throttle. We didn't know each other, but Cristina had heard that I would be up for an adventure. She invited me to be her partner for the 2014 International South Beach Triathlon. I needed little persuasion. We chose our team's name, ThumbsUp, to reflect my signature gesture.

Our joint participation created so much momentum and support that the two of us were encouraged to cofound a nonprofit and organize efforts for others, both disabled and able-bodied so that others could have the same joyous, empowering, life-changing experience. With the help of a group of enthusiastic fellow able-bodied triathletes, ThumbsUp International was formed. The expanded name reflects the nonprofit foundation's ambitions to spread its wings around the world. Since then, I have continued to compete in endurance races with different partners, even finishing Ironman Florida in 2015 with Caryn Lubetsky, an able-bodied athlete.

Most satisfying, however, is seeing the organization, which was born out of Cristina's impulse, grow and flourish. Like all startups, it has had some challenges, but more importantly, it has had a positive effect on people of all abilities. But I maintain that its most profound impact has been personal. I have learned so much about myself: my strengths and gifts, deficits and weaknesses. I've learned what's important and what I need to let go of; where I should focus my energy and talents; what I need to admit isn't my forte; and especially that we need to be responsible for changing ourselves first before we can effectively change others. I see this as a new beginning, another door opening, another opportunity. It is definitely a process. So the journey continues, with my deep gratitude to Cristina for her kindness and trust in me.

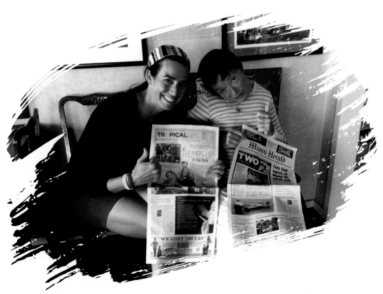

Kerry with Cristina spreading the word about ThumbsUp International.

Addendum
By Cristina Ramirez

Kindness can often best express itself when someone really needs help. Kerry embodies this fact, and she told me so directly. Kerry needs help with every single daily activity. She doesn't see that as a burden but has learned to see it as a gift. When someone is able to help her with anything…whether it's as big as a running with her in a triathlon race or as small as pushing her wheelchair for daily tasks, that person feels great to have been able to help someone who really needs the help.

If Kerry didn't need all that help, she wouldn't be so impactful in her message and so generous in her ability to give others an opportunity to feel good by doing something helpful. She would simply do these things by herself, to the best of her ability, as the rest of us do. If she could do a triathlon by herself, she would! But then I and many others would not have been touched by the experience of helping her push her limits. And boy, are we ever so touched.

Love you, Kerry!

"To love oneself is to love life. It is essential to understand that we make ourselves happy in making others happy."

—*Matthieu Ricard*

Marathon Mate
By Rochelle Baer

I was invited to be part of the Miami Marathon 2015 with ThumbsUp International, a nonprofit organization that matches able-bodied athletes with individuals with disabilities to participate in sporting events. It was a strange time for me—my father had passed away three weeks before. I wasn't sure I wanted to be part of the marathon. But then I thought of my dad, and I knew that he would have wanted me to have this experience. He was always my biggest cheerleader. So I said yes, knowing nothing at all about the athlete I would be matched with.

The day before the race I was outfitted with a chair resembling a cross between a stroller and a wheelchair. The runner would push me in it, and I would remain seated. Because I was going to be sitting, I was advised to dress warmly. I had to borrow a ski-type jacket from my neighbor as it was predicted to be cold—yes, it can occasionally get cold in Miami!

My husband dropped me off at 4 a.m. at Bayfront Park. It was so early that I was barely conscious. Making matters worse was the fact that I skipped my usual morning coffee. I couldn't even remember why I wanted to participate in this event. But then I met my two pushers—two women, a lovely couple from nearby, who seemed far too bubbly for that early-morning hour. We exchanged small talk until it was time to head to the starting line.

Waiting among the throngs of thousands of runners of all shapes, ages and sizes for the gun to signal the start of the race, the energy and enthusiasm were palpable. I felt teary and dizzy and part of it all, decked out in my bright-blue souvenir marathon T-shirt. For the next few hours, my two runners alternated pushing me, keeping a steady pace.

And then the most amazing thing happened.

About an hour before the end of the race, a woman who introduced herself as Ahuva offered to assist my runners in pushing me. She could tell they were tired and just took over—which the couple was glad to let her do. Ahuva and I got to talking, and immediately we clicked. We got on so well that she pushed me for the rest of the race, which meant she sacrificed a faster race time.

We discovered we had much in common. Ahuva was an Orthodox Jewish woman from New York City who had flown down for the marathon—she flies many places to run. She had gone to Yeshiva University for her master's degree in social work, just as I had. I told her about my dad, and we cried together. I loved her ease and energy and her ability to speak with anyone, even strangers. I could barely see her throughout the race—I could only hear her singsong voice and feel the thud of her sneakers hitting the ground.

Ahuva ran me over the finish line. She transported me, literally, beyond my pain, if just for a moment. I felt dizzy with awe when my marathon medal was placed over my head. It was all so exciting. And I was glad to have met Ahuva, my new friend.

> "One thing I know: the only ones among you who will be really happy are those who will have sought and found how to serve."
>
> —Albert Schweitzer

Metro North
By Amy Kalafa

The 5:35 p.m. train was crowded by the time I got on. I was relieved to be heading home to Connecticut after my first day back in the city since 9/11. It hadn't gone well. Every sound was amplified; every siren jolted me. Three weeks earlier, I had borne witness to the events of that day and I was still feeling pretty traumatized.

I don't like sitting in those face-to-face sections where knees collide and you're forced to be social, but the train was filling fast and this looked to be my best option. A touristy looking couple took up two of the six seats. I sat down in the window seat of the empty row across from them. As I was settling in, a young woman hastily plunked herself down on the end seat and gingerly placed a small carrying case on the seat between us. She unzipped the bag's cover and pulled out a limp and shaggy white dog with dirty matted fur. She gently placed the meek little moppy thing on the middle seat and stowed the case above us. Over the course of the next several minutes, a man in a business suit grabbed the remaining seat, and our little compartment was filled with five humans and a sleeping dog.

Latecomers, seeing what looked like an open seat, scowled when they saw the little pup taking up a coveted spot. I, too, was feeling resentful of the bedraggled beast. Its owner, however, sat blissfully unaware, softly patting his little head, oblivious to the glares of the passersby. The critic in me started analyzing. Her perfectly coiffed auburn hair, matching purse and shoes and careful make-up suggested a tony corporate life. Surely such a woman should have a canine companion that reflected her upscale style.

The scorn with which I regarded the petite woman and the pathetic creature that lay splayed between us was a welcome distraction from the terrifying flashbacks I'd experienced all day. What kind of privilege did she feel entitled this dirty pup to its own seat?

As the train pulled out of the station, the tourist couple smiled benevolently at the dog. The older woman spoke up. "He's so cute. What kind of dog is he?"

My seatmate smiled back, and answered, "I'm not sure. We think maybe Lhasa Apso? I'm just fostering him. The owner worked in the Towers and never made it home. A neighbor was able to get in after ten days and rescue this little guy. Nobody knows how he managed to survive all that time."

I felt the blood rush to my face and tears well in my eyes. The businessman looked up from his newspaper and smiled. I suddenly realized that these kindly tourists were some of the first fearless visitors venturing to New York City in solidarity. With my self-absorbed, judgmental indignation brought to heel by the story of this woman's act of kindness, for the first time in weeks I felt safe. I was united with a community of caring souls. The sad little shaggy dog and his caregiver had helped me see that in order to heal from my own trauma, I needed to re-engage and be open to the world around me.

"The greatness of a nation and its moral progress can be measured by the way its animals are treated."
—Mahatma Gandhi

Teeing Off
By Ian Shapiro

It was a bright sunny day, not unlike most other Florida days. I was scheduled to play in a golf tournament at the Doral, which is about an hour away from where I live and a bit farther from my practice course. I was feeling calm and excited and was focused on playing my best. My dad normally accompanies me to tournaments but he had a complicated legal case he needed to handle. My dad is a criminal defense attorney, and I have found it best not to ask him exactly what he is working on. I just need to understand that he can't accompany me all the time.

I knew it would only be another year before I got my driver's license, and this problem would be solved. My mother passed away after a long battle with cancer, so it was just me and Dad in the house, and I knew at times I had to do my best to take care of myself. My game had slumped when Mom got sick. Two years had passed without Mom, and I was trying hard to get my game back on track. I knew it meant a lot to my dad. He had been a quarterback at the University of North Carolina, and we shared the dream that I would also play a sport in college.

My dad first took me golfing when I was four, and I was hooked almost immediately. He coached and caddied for me, and I won a lot of tournaments. But after I lost my mom, everything changed. Today was an important day to me, to my dad and I hoped to my mom. I knew she would be sad to see how her loss was impacting me.

I went out for a few practice rounds before the match and was playing alone. The young woman in front of me was also playing alone and was a bit slow, so I asked if I could join her. I was never one to be shy. We played the next few holes together, and she seemed quite nice. She asked me about school, my family and golf, and I offered her a few pointers which she seemed to appreciate. I enjoyed the company, as it helped me calm my nerves before my start time.

On the eighth hole, playing from the back tee in what was by that time blazing sun, my swing was a bit off, and my ball ended up in the water. Already sweating from the heat, I felt a new rush of water pour down my back. I didn't have another ball. The truth is, I rarely lost one, and I had rushed out when my Uber arrived a few minutes earlier than I had expected. Panic came over me. As you may know, golf is a game of nerves and this certainly wasn't going to help mine.

I knew this wasn't the best golf etiquette, but I really had no option, so when my new golf partner handed me a ball, I grabbed it and placed it on the tee. As I began to swing, I got distracted by something on the ball. I stopped and bent down to pick it up. To my great surprise, I saw my dad's name on it. It was a ball that I had given him last Father's Day. I'd bought him a box of twelve balls with his name on them, and he had been very pleased with the gift. He plays often, but at a course nowhere near where we were playing. He rarely loses balls as his game is even better than mine.

How did his ball get here? How did this woman have it? Why did I ask this woman if I could join her? How did I lose my ball? These and a thousand other questions swirled through my mind, but I knew it was time to focus.

I birdied the next hole, which means I shot really well (for you non-golfers!) and then it was time to begin the tournament. I thanked the woman, who was also quite surprised by this remarkable coincidence, and I ran off. I finished first for the first time in three years, and I thanked my kind golf mate for getting me out of my slump.

I continue to practice every day and have started to meet with college coaches, and I am once again feeling like I can live the dream that my dad and I created so many years ago.

The Golden Rule

The world's major religions share many guiding principles, including what is referred to as The Golden Rule, "Do unto others as you would have them do unto you." (New Testament, Matthew 7:12). British theologians popularized The Golden Rule in the early seventeenth century, but the concept originated as early as 2040 BC in Egypt: "Do to the doer to make him do." Confucius in 500 BC said, "Never impose on others what you would not choose for yourself."

At the Parliament of the World's Religions, a global interfaith movement, over 8,000 people from across the globe gathered in Chicago in 1993 to celebrate, discuss and explore how people from different religious traditions can work together on the critical issues which confront the world. They proclaimed The Golden Rule as their common guiding principle, reminding us that our core religious beliefs share deeply held ethical principles. While entire libraries have been written on this theme, here is a very brief look at the ways that some religious faiths express the concept of The Golden Rule:

Buddhism: Hurt not others in ways that you yourself would find hurtful.

Baha'i: Blessed are those who prefer others before themselves.

Christianity: Do unto others as you would have them do unto you.

Jainism: In happiness and suffering, in joy and grief, regard all creatures as you would your own self.

Judaism: What is hateful to you do not do to your neighbor. That is the entire Torah. The rest is commentary, go learn.

Islam: No one is a believer until you desire for another that which you desire for yourself.

Sikhism: Be not estranged from one another, for God dwells in every heart.

Zoroastrianism: Human nature is good only when it does not do unto another whatever is not good for its own self.

Women of Tomorrow
By Nathalie Mora

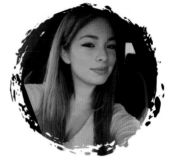

I am 21 years old, in college and working full time, all due to the kindness of three women who have taken me under their wings. They are always happy to help me. We meet for coffee often. I share with them my family problems. These women have totally changed my life.

I grew up in South Miami area. My home life was not so great. My mom works cleaning houses, and my dad is a mechanic for a plant nursery. My dad is Cuban, and my mom is from Guatemala. I struggled since the beginning of school because even though I was born in the U.S., I didn't learn English until third grade.

My freshman year at Palmetto High School, I was doing very poorly and skipping a lot of classes. I never did drugs, but my brother got into cocaine, and I saw how it destroyed my family. My mom tries to be the best mom, but she is stressed by my brother. She tries to help him, but nothing seems to work.

One day I was walking into the library, and a friend asked me if I could go with her to a meeting. I saw cookies and cupcakes, so I said sure. I asked what it was, and she said it was a meeting called "Women of Tomorrow."

I came to learn that the Women of Tomorrow Mentor & Scholarship Program is a group of accomplished professional women who mentor small groups of girls in public high schools. Each month, a different speaker comes to teach and motivate us. We learn how to relax, to meditate, to shake a person's hand, to look them in the eye, and how to write a resume. I took in everything they said and tried to ignore what was going on in my home life. Things started getting better and better until one day when my dad and brother got in a fight that turned violent. I was so shaken up. I started missing school again. I wouldn't talk to anyone. I sat alone, and I was very depressed.

The Women of Tomorrow mentors talked to me and made me feel better. They emailed the teachers saying that I had family issues and please excuse any absences. Girls from the Women of Tomorrow program came to see me, and they became my support system.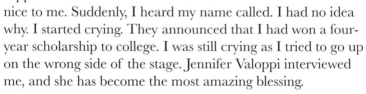

Five days after the incident at home, I was sitting at a luncheon, eating chocolate cake and yawning. I was a bit bored but had gone to support the women that had been so nice to me. Suddenly, I heard my name called. I had no idea why. I started crying. They announced that I had won a four-year scholarship to college. I was still crying as I tried to go up on the wrong side of the stage. Jennifer Valoppi interviewed me, and she has become the most amazing blessing.

Jennifer asked me to dog sit for her, and since I want to be a veterinarian, I jumped at the offer. I am now at Miami Dade College, where the scholarship has paid for everything. Jennifer got me a tutor for chemistry, and I am doing really well. After this summer, I will transfer to Florida International University and go into the pre-veterinary program there and, I am excited to continue on the path that the Women of Tomorrow Mentors helped me find.

Multiplied Blessings
By Reverend Carolyn McCombs

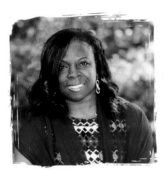

I have the privilege of serving as director of New Destiny
Family Success Center, a neighborhood-based family support
center in the Great Falls section of downtown Paterson, New
Jersey's third-largest city. Paterson is a melting pot of people
from over eighty nations. Many of the individuals are brand
new to the shores of the United States, and a substantial
number are also working families. Many are of African-
American descent, whose ancestors migrated to Paterson from
the South back in the 1950s and '60s. Paterson is plagued with
issues of unemployment, struggling schools, poverty and many
other ills that affect a post-industrial city.

New Destiny's mission, in the midst of our challenging
environment, is to inspire hope and faith in Paterson's families
to thrive and prosper. We are not a typical social-service agency
offering our perspective on what families should do to address
their needs; instead, we are like partners who offer listening
ears, advocacy and access to resources to help families navigate
their challenges. We believe that every family has strengths
and, as they tap into their own strengths, they feel empowered
and equipped to move forward to prosperity.

Our funding partner at the State of New Jersey (the
Department of Children and Families) has directed each

Family Success Center to reevaluate its physical space, making sure it has a home-like look and feel. Of course, this recommendation comes without any additional funding, but with a strong directive to creatively look at ways to get it done without additional resources. At our recent staff meeting in early December, our team began to think about ways to rearrange our space to reflect this new home-like mood. Needless to say, while we were willing to do our best, our efforts would be constrained by our lack of resources.

About a week after the staff meeting, I had the opportunity to catch up with a friend and colleague, Patrice Samara. After our brief chat, with me mostly sharing my latest dilemma, Patrice began to reflect on a challenge she was having selling her home in Connecticut. I could hear in her voice her sorrow over having to give away or throw away some of her most cherished family possessions (including furniture, fine china and wall fixtures), which she'd accumulated over the years.

A light bulb went off in my head. I told Patrice, "It is interesting that our team was just discussing how we would meet the state's latest requirement to give a home-like look and feel to our space. This would be extremely difficult to do without funds, and we need the furniture, fixtures and artwork that you find in a typical house."

Instantly, I heard a sigh of relief, excitement, and catch in her throat. Patrice's offered: "I don't need to sell these items; I just need to know that they will be put to good use and that someone else could gain some enjoyment from my cherished family possessions."

It was a perfect match: we had a need, and Patrice could fill it! Yes, it was a win-win. As if this weren't enough, Patrice shared that her friend, Deborah, an accomplished NYC interior designer, wanted to donate her talents to create an inviting space for immigrant women and victims of domestic violence. We now had a win-win-win. Not only would our center become the recipient of this huge blessing from Patrice, but we would have the generous expertise of a professional designer to bring everything together to create a warm, inviting retreat for the troubled souls who enter our doors.

Deborah also began reaching out to her contacts in the field for donations of paint, fabrics, supplies and other essentials. Suddenly, there were more and more generous donors.

A friend of Patrice's, Joyce, believed in *hesed*. *Hesed* is one of the most profound words in the Old Testament. *Hesed* is not primarily something that people "feel." It is something that people "do" for other people without expectation of reward. *Hesed* is often translated as kindness. Joyce also made a very generous donation of furnishings that complemented Patrice and Deborah's.

From Patrice's one random act of kindness, we have had a crescendo of blessings that will benefit hundreds of women, youth and families. The moment they step through our warm, newly designed space, they will know…and feel…that someone took the time to make sure they felt welcomed and valued. It has become a win-win-win-win!

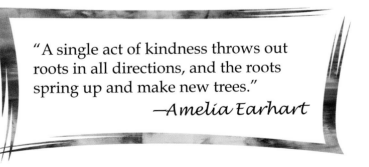

"A single act of kindness throws out roots in all directions, and the roots spring up and make new trees."
—Amelia Earhart

Can Kindness Extend Your Life?

Yes, it can! Sara Konrath, Ph.D. of the University of Michigan looked at 10,317 Wisconsin residents and asked how often they had volunteered in the last ten years. The study found that those who volunteered for altruistic reasons had lower mortality rates than those who did not: 1.6 percent vs. 4.3 percent mortality within four years.

This data makes sense given what we learned about the health benefits of oxytocin. We know that feeling close to others allows us to release more of it and improves our health. The national volunteer rate was 24.9 percent for the year ending in September 2015, according to the U.S. Bureau of Labor Statistics. About 62.6 million people volunteered through or for an organization at least once between September 2014 and September 2015. Volunteers are defined as persons who did unpaid work (except for expenses) through or for an organization. We are a kind nation!

© Masha Melnik

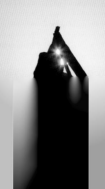

The volunteer rate for men was 21.8 percent, and the rate for women was 27.8 percent. Across all age groups, educational levels and other major demographic characteristics, women continued to volunteer at a higher rate than men. Thirty-five- to 44-year-olds and 45- to 54-year-olds were the most likely to volunteer (28.9 percent and 28.0 percent, respectively). Volunteer rates were lowest among 20- to 24-year-olds (18.4 percent).

Why is one out of every four people willing to give up his or her time to help others? "Helper's high" and "giver's glow" are terms used to describe the positive emotional state some people experience after providing help to others, and it is the pursuit of those feelings that drives so many of us to volunteer. Studies have shown that helping others can produce feelings of happiness and can activate reward centers of the brain just like food, sex and drugs.

According to brain scans, the mere thought of helping others by planning to make a donation makes people happier. Such thoughts activate the mesolimbic pathway in the brain that is associated with happiness and production of dopamine, a neurotransmitter that helps control the brain's reward and pleasure centers. Actual face-to-face helping also triggers areas of the brain associated with happiness.

"It is one of the beautiful compensations of life that no man can sincerely help another without helping himself."
—Ralph Waldo Emerson

Our Wonderful World
By Jimena Stein

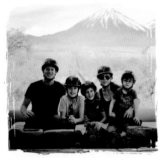

One morning about a year ago, I found myself immersed in the news that depicted a scary world. I was taking a warm shower and thought, "I am so glad we traveled when we did and not now." I then stopped myself, realizing I had fallen prey to fear and to the media that chooses to highlight the negative realities of our world. I reminded myself that during our journey we had never once felt afraid; on the contrary, we often felt inspired and humbled by the evidence of kindness that permeates our world. Let me explain.

On June 18, 2014, my husband, our three boys and I embarked on the adventure of a lifetime. In order to spend more time with our sons, who seemed to be growing up so fast, we decided to take a year off of our hectic lives and travel around the world together. We had pulled our children out of school, taken sabbaticals from our jobs and packed our bags. After a year of planning, the day finally came, and we were ready to board our first flight of many.

The final tally came to seventy-three flights and eighty-one places we stayed—from hotels to safari camps, small family-owned inns to cruise ships and rainforest lodges. We fell in love with our planet thanks to all of those who along the way helped us see the world through their eyes.

What we experienced was so extraordinary it's hard to put into words. Not just because of the things we saw, but also for the kindness we experienced. You see, during our journey, we found nothing but welcoming faces, eager smiles, curious eyes and nods of acknowledgment, whether in small villages not to be found on maps or in large metropolises like Shanghai and Tokyo.

Kindness has a loud presence in our world. We heard it in the story of the doctor we met in Zambia. He had originally traveled there with the intention of working for only a couple of months but ended up adopting the child of one of his patients who had succumbed to HIV/AIDS and stayed on. We saw it in the story of the South African family, who, despite having very little resources of their own, served as an adoptive family and transition home for ten children.

In Zimbabwe, a country where a dictatorship has destroyed its economy and left millions destitute, kindness rang loud because of an organization, made possible by a generous foreign philanthropist, that provides over twenty thousand daily breakfasts of porridge in just one town. And in Amman, 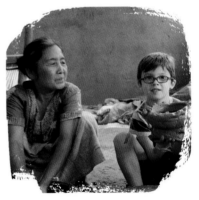 Jordan, we were lucky to meet an American woman with a passion for empowering females, who had just moved her whole family to the country to run a program that promised to see Jordanian women rise.

The stories of kindness followed one after another. And many challenged the models and rules we live by. For example, in Myanmar, we learned that the tradition is to give on your birthday, instead of receiving gifts. My son, who turned twelve

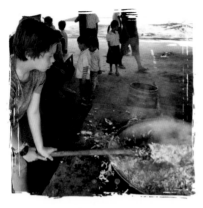

during our time there, embraced that tradition by donating and serving lunch to sixty-eight Buddhist monks and novices on his birthday.

During those thirteen months, I experienced our common humanity. Yes, we saw firsthand a world that shares a history of cruelty, war, oppression, poverty and injustice. But those problems were drowned out by stories of sacrifice, heroic accounts of nations that overcame adversity and tales of kindness that transcends borders making us deeply appreciative of our wonderful world.

"But perhaps human kindness is like air: We constantly move within it and can easily forget entirely that it is there. Only when we're deprived of it do we realize what we are missing."

—Stefan Klein, Ph.D.
Survival of the Nicest

The Currency of Kindness
By Marly Q. Casanova

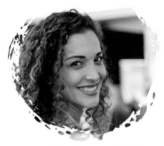

When I think of kindness, I'm immediately reminded of my 4th grade teacher, Ms. Giro, and the day my class went on a field trip to clean up the park. Most kids were happy to ditch school, but not me. I was so excited to help the environment, like my favorite superhero, Captain Planet. Unfortunately, this field trip wasn't free and, at that time, my parents couldn't afford it.

I was heartbroken as my classmates boarded the bus.

Ms. Giro noticed and gently whispered in my ear to step aside as the other children were leaving for the field trip. I began crying as I expressed how upset I was to not have enough money to go and make a difference. She stopped me, looked right in my eyes and said: "You don't need money to make a difference." She told me I was the kindest kid she's ever met and that my smile brightened up her day. She noted I held the door open for others, lent my supplies and always asked how I could help. Ms. Giro taught me that the currency of kindness is more important than the currency of money.

She said kindness is my superpower…and from that day forward, I believed her! I've carried this lesson with me my entire life. I'm still amazed at how such simple words could have such a profound and lasting ripple effect.

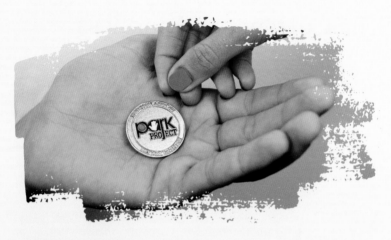

Postscript: In 2010, fifteen years later, Marly Q. Casanova founded **PARK Project**, a nonprofit organization on a mission to inspire people to "Perform Acts of Random Kindness" worldwide. This volunteer-driven movement is made up of kind people who are making the world a better place by donating their valuable time, energy and enthusiasm. They are using SPARK Coins, as the currency of kindness. These coins contain a unique platform and code that tracks the ripple effect as it is passed from person to person. Users can share kind stories on social media using #wePARK.

"Act as if what you do makes a difference. It does."

—*William James*

Adoption

The ultimate act of kindness? Some might say it's adoption. What could Bekindr than taking someone into your home and feeding, clothing and educating them for close to two decades? About 135,000 children are adopted in the United States each year. Of non-stepparent adoptions, about 59 percent are from the child welfare (or foster) system, 26 percent are from other countries and 15 percent are voluntarily relinquished American babies.

This act of kindness is one that profoundly alters both the giver and the receiver. The process of becoming a parent is tremendously life-altering. I mentioned oxytocin earlier. It is released when you are close to someone, and it allows you to literally rewire your brain. Nature in her inimitable wisdom has created the perfect system. A small dependent creature comes into your life, your brain secretes chemicals that allow you to rewire, and the next thing you know, their needs come before yours. We can activate this same system when we fall in love and get close to another adult or animal as well. Nothing feels better than falling in love because nothing is as important to our survival.

© Kate Luber

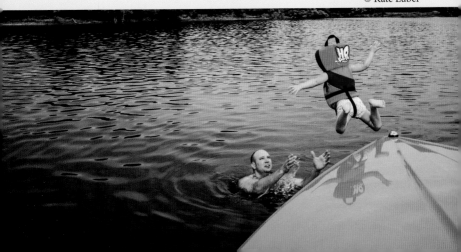

Eighteen Seconds
By Cheryl Carter Shotts

I was home watching *60 Minutes* and had no idea that 18 seconds were about to change my life. I saw Diane Sawyer interview a boy in the West African country of Mali, and lightning struck.

"Where do you sleep?" she asked. "Here," he said. "On the ground?" she continued. "Yes," he answered. "Are you hungry?" "Yes," he said. "All the time?" she asked. "Yes, many childrens they are dead." "You have seen many children die?" Diane asked. "Yes," the boy confirmed.

For the next three nights, as I would try to fall asleep, I asked my husband, "Do you think that little boy has eaten today?" On the fourth morning, I told my husband, "I don't understand, but that boy is my son and I have to find my son and bring him home."

I knew nothing about Africa, about international adoption, and nothing about the boy—I just knew I had to bring him home. I quit my work and devoted every waking minute to finding him. I wrote Diane Sawyer through her secretary. Ms. Sawyer called, and we spoke for an hour. "He is handicapped—did you know that? He was alone with no family," Diane volunteered. None of that deterred me.

My husband and I maxed out our credit cards, used our savings and borrowed $7,000 so he could head off to the Sahara Desert and find our son.

On December 7, 1985, Mohammed stepped off a plane in Indianapolis with his new father, and into my arms. He was 5'4" tall, weighed 65 pounds and was head to toe medical problems. He looked about 9 or 10 years old but doctors estimated he was 13 or 14.

Mohammed thought he had been brought to America to be my "house boy." When I explained that he had been brought to the U.S. to be my son, he said he didn't know what that meant but said, "If you will teach me, I promise to learn."

Within days Mohammed was talking about his friend, Nimit, who was left behind in the Sahara. He wanted Nimit to have a family, too. I decided that I had to help other African children, and the idea for Americans for African Adoptions, Inc. (AFAA) was born. To date, AFAA has brought 765 African orphans from Mali, Liberia, Sierra Leone, Ethiopia, Uganda, Lesotho, and three special needs children from Mogadishu, Somalia, to new families across the U.S., Canada and New Zealand.

Because of those 18 seconds, Mohammed is a healthy adult. Five major surgeries rebuilt his body and on May 23, 1998, Mohammed graduated from the School of Foreign Service at Georgetown University, with *Dateline* on hand for a second momentous time in his life. Today, he is a husband and a father. He speaks six languages and works for the U.S. government in Washington, D.C. Each year, we celebrate his birthday on August 11, the day I first saw him on *60 Minutes*.

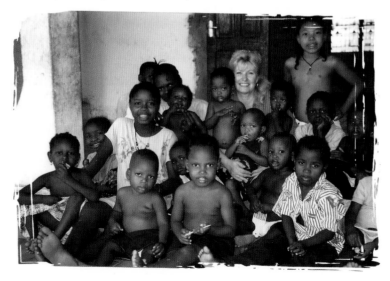

The Operator
By Anne Bielamowicz

When I was a teenager, I longed for adventure. Although I came from a close-knit family, I left my home in California to attend a boarding school in England. The year brought all I had hoped—adventure, excitement and independence, but also one tremendous scare. My father, an active, energetic, fit man in his late forties, suffered a serious heart attack. I was home with him on my spring break at the time it occurred but had to fly back to England to finish the year while he was still in the hospital.

Shortly after his heart attack, he underwent quadruple bypass surgery. This surgery is pretty scary today. Forty years ago, it was cutting edge and terrifying. There is an eight-hour time difference between London and Los Angeles so the surgery took place around midnight my time. I was desperate for information. I found a payphone on a street corner in London and—this was a LONG time ago—reached an operator who helped me place a call to the United States. I was a 15-year-old girl alone in an alley in London. I was petrified.

The call to my house was unsuccessful, and the operator said goodnight to me and was about to disconnect. Then he paused and asked me if I was okay. I explained the situation. His warmth and kindness wrapped around me in a bear hug. He assured me he would stay on the phone with me until we knew my dad was okay. He called the hospital and persisted in working his way through the convoluted chain all the while talking to me, keeping me calm, assuring me I was not alone.

That call took place ages ago, but I can still recall the sense of relief I had when we finally reached home. My dad was okay. That operator became family to me that night. I knew he would take care of me…and he did.

Reborn
By Ed Ritvo

Years after my multiple heart attacks and bypass surgery, my heart gave out. I was 69 years old. There was only one option left.

Inert, flat on my back, chest cut open from neck to belly button, my heart in a tin bucket by my feet. Call it what you want: I call it dead.

Then a cheer I could not hear rose through the doctors and nurses hovering over me, who were pumping blood through my chilled corpse.

"They're here!"

In rushed a second team of doctors and nurses, just off a helicopter that had bounced down onto the roof of Cedars Sinai Hospital two minutes earlier. The helicopter had met a private jet at the Los Angeles airport—it had just arrived from Seattle three minutes before.

Dangling in the hand of an angel I couldn't see was a little "Eskimo" cooler, and inside that was the ultimate gift: a human heart. Dr. Blanch opened the cooler as gently as possible and lifted the trembling heart from within. He bathed it in a special elixir and lowered it into my empty chest. Would it beat? Had it been in flight too long? Would it match my body size? These and a thousand other questions raced through the minds and hearts of those crowded around.

You see, a young man in his mid-twenties had died that morning in a motorcycle crash outside Seattle. That's all I know about him. His mother, a brave soul, knew that she would have to live with the tragedy of his sudden death for the rest of her life—but she also knew that she could spare others the tragedy of losing a loved one by donating her son's organs. And she had the wisdom and courage to do so.

Dr. Blanch sewed in the new heart and applied a small electric pulse. The ultimate gift started beating. And it has been beating for sixteen years in its new home, my chest. I was no longer dead.

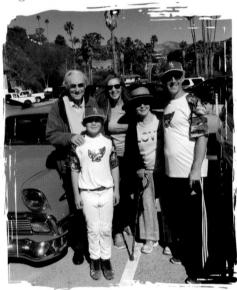

These sixteen years have been a gift of life, cherished and appreciated every day, through good and bad. I returned to parenting my children, to my medical and research career, to the joy of seeing grandchildren born and the tragedy of cancer taking my youngest son.

People ask, "What does it feel like to have someone else's heart beating in your chest? Does it make you feel different?"

My answer is, "I feel like my old self, but this experience is different from any other." To know that my heart transplant required someone's death is an experience of such magnitude I don't have words to describe it. It is the rule of the transplant committee that I do not learn any details of my donor's life. I respect that.

But I am indebted to his courageous mother in a way that only someone in such debt can truly appreciate. I bless her every day and thank her son for this heart—the ultimate gift.

What if Kindness Goes Wrong?

H ow many of us have loaned money and not gotten it back? Or given money to a homeless man only to see him an hour later with a bottle in his hand? Or done a simple thing like holding a door open for someone who fails to express gratitude for our gesture?

It's important not to be deterred by these negative outcomes. The error was not in the act of kindness. As they say in Alcoholic Anonymous: "Keep your side of the street clean." In life, you are only responsible for yourself and your children. As long as you operate to the highest of your ability with kindness, compassion and integrity, you can sleep soundly at night knowing your side of the street is clean. Often, the outcome is out of our hands.

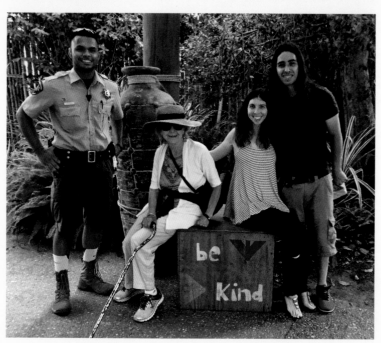

Strangers' Blood
By Jenna Jagodzinska

Thirty-six weeks into my third pregnancy, I was diagnosed with placenta accreta, which is when your placenta grows through the wall of your uterus. There was a chance it was attached to my bladder, and it was likely I would need a hysterectomy after a C-section to deliver my son. It was a horrible shock, as I was very healthy and had had two easy pregnancies. Thankfully, it was diagnosed by a brilliant sonographer at my last scan, who called me back in to double check. She was the first person who helped save my life! If it had gone undiagnosed and I'd had a routine C-section, there would have been a much greater chance of fatal blood loss.

I had an elective C-section on January 20, 2015. My husband and father were with me. I was in great hands at Derriford Hospital in Plymouth, where my husband and I had both worked (I as a physiotherapist, he as a surgeon). I felt pretty calm and positive about it, but I think my family was terrified. I was expected to lose a lot of blood, and they had booked me a bed in the intensive therapy unit.

I needed thirteen units of blood products during my C-section. When I came round, my first question was if my son was okay. Zak was a healthy six pounds, five ounces, and was being looked after by the nurses. My second question was if they had had to resect my bladder. Fortunately, they hadn't, as the placenta wasn't attached to it, but they'd had to perform a hysterectomy to stop the bleeding. I didn't care. I had two healthy kids, and I was going to be okay. Or so I thought…

Two days later I was rushed back to the hospital with internal bleeding. They drained nearly one and a half gallons of blood from my abdomen. I received another twenty-two units of blood and blood products. I remember asking the nurse as they took me to the operating theater if they had enough blood for me, and she was very reassuring. Back to ITU (Intensive Treatment Unit) I went! I made a good recovery, and Zak and I were home within eight days. I'd had over three times my circulating blood volume replaced, the equivalent of thirty-three separate blood and platelet donations. Perhaps thirty-three total strangers each gave a bit of their blood one day (on their lunch break, with a friend, after school or on the weekend). That blood was given to me in theater, pumped through my body and my heart, and it kept me alive. I went home from the hospital holding my gorgeous boy, and none of the blood in my body was mine! I felt pretty lucky.

I can't ever thank those strangers whose blood I received. But to anyone out there who does something as brilliant and selfless as giving blood: you saved my life. That's how it feels to me. You are superheroes.

I can't give blood anymore, as I've had multiple transfusions. So in order to try and give some blood back, I asked my friends on Facebook to donate blood. My brilliant and lovely friends gave over one hundred donations the next year. I did a bit of media work for Give Blood U.K. to raise awareness and try a encourage people to give blood. In the United Kingdom, 5 percent of the population gives blood, but 60 percent could. Such a simple gift saves lives.

"Compassion is a verb."

—Thich Nhat Hanh,
Vietnamese Zen Monk

A Chance Meeting
By Anonymous

I was raised in an upper-middle-class family in Cuba. My father was one of the deans of the University of Havana, my mother had a Ph.D. in sociology, and we lived well. After high school, I went to college and spent six years studying to become a doctor. Following medical school, I spent another four years training in family medicine. Finally, I was done with my education. I had a good life ahead of me in Cuba, but there was one problem: I was gay.

Being gay in Cuba at that time was not acceptable, and I was scared that someone would find out, and I would be in danger. I decided I needed to leave.

I was able to get into the United States on a tourist visa and decided to go to Miami since I had a lot of family members there. I moved in with my aunt and was trying to pass the medical board licensing in order to be able to practice in the U.S.

The exams are very difficult, so I needed time to study and learn English. I had no money. After working several months as a waiter, I got a job cleaning a house for a man my cousin knew. I began working for him and was relieved to have a stable income. He asked me many questions while I was there. One day as I was leaving, he gave me an envelope and told me not to come back. I had a sinking feeling, as I thought I'd been fired. When I got to my car, I opened the envelope and found a check for $5,000. I was elated! After receiving that gift, I was able to spend all day and night learning English and studying for the medical board.

I returned to thank the man, and we became friends. Soon after, we began dating. He introduced me to a world I had only seen in the movies: We traveled throughout the U.S. and I was exposed to many new things. We were in love and happy. We moved in together, and I was grateful to have the opportunity to dedicate all of my time to studying medicine.

However, as the months passed, things between us declined. He was a drinker, and his alcohol use started to interfere in our relationship. One night, he failed to come home at all. In the morning, I told him if it ever happened again, I would leave. Soon after, he did it again. Though I loved him and had learned so much during my time with him, I just didn't feel I could continue in a relationship under these conditions.

We remained friends, and he got in a new relationship.

Three months after I left, he called to tell me that he was going to give me the building where we had been living. I remember his exact words: "This will be your retirement plan." He moved out, and I moved back in.

I went on to pass the test. I was accepted into a residency training program and was finally able to begin the life I had worked so hard to achieve.

Twenty-one years have passed since I first came to the U.S. I have a busy medical practice and am so grateful to be living in Miami in the building that was given to me so many years ago. This chance meeting changed my life immediately and continues to impact me every day. I don't know what my life would have been like if we hadn't met that day in the summer of 1995, but I do know it wouldn't be the way it is now.

> "Three things in human life are important. The first is to be kind. The second is to be kind. And the third is to be kind."
>
> —Henry James

Flower Boutique
By Eduardo Martinez

As soon as she walked in, he felt the tension. She reminded him of a bird with a broken wing who was determined to fly. He shuddered as a look of curiosity and respect fought behind his mask of humility.

While she moved through the small flower boutique, silently admiring the colorful flowers blossoming in his endangered establishment, he politely asked, "May I help you, young lady?"

She replied, "I saw these white baby roses from outside. They're enchanting!" Her eyes reminded him of the day after Christmas, a wintery one, and he wondered what could possibly be troubling this beautiful young woman, this star that seemed to have fallen. She obviously needed space, so he gave her a galaxy. After all, that's where all stars reside.

He watched her carefully. She nobly greeted every flower with appreciation, enjoyed every distinct fragrance and gave each one a chance to welcome her. Finally, she worked her way over to the small wooden counter and inquired about the white baby roses with the light peach-tipped petals.

He said, "Young lady, for you, twenty roses for five dollars cash."

She reached into her small purse, removed a five-dollar bill, handed it to him and thanked him. He accepted it with a smile and asked her with playful charm, "Aren't you a day late? Valentine's Day was yesterday. Shouldn't a lucky young man be buying you flowers?"

She paused for a second as if considering whether or not to answer his question. She grabbed her flowers and replied, "My husband is in prison. I just left from visiting him…and if my husband was home, he wouldn't give me roses. He'd give me a garden."

The old man apologized and understood immediately. For he, too, had once been imprisoned and in love. He watched as she walked out of his boutique and headed toward her car.

As she was opening her door, she turned her head when the old man yelled, "Young lady, young lady. Wait! You forgot these."

He held another twenty-five roses in his hand. She looked confused. The old man smiled. "These are from your husband."

The young lady's smile opened like a sunflower correcting the morning sun. She thanked the old man with tears in her eyes.

As she got into her car with the roses, she remembered her birthday a few months ago. Her husband had sent her a bouquet of flowers, a small box of chocolate and a cute little card. She blushed as she remembered what he had written: "My love, I couldn't wait to show these flowers how pretty you are."

She wiped a tearful diamond off her cheek. Dropped tension off in the parking lot of the small boutique. Picked up patience and drove off with fifty envious roses.

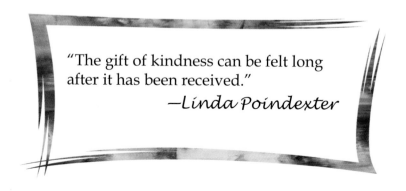

"The gift of kindness can be felt long after it has been received."
—Linda Poindexter

The Miracle of the Butterfly
By Valeria Geritzen

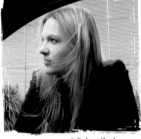

When I was a little girl in Germany and visiting my grandma, I found a butterfly trapped behind her kitchen window. Even though I was very young, I was aware of my power to free the beautiful creature. I told my grandma and, together, we beheld its beauty briefly. Then we carefully removed the obstacles in front of the window and gently opened it. The butterfly was gone in a second. Soon after, guests arrived for afternoon coffee and cake and in my little girl's mind, it seemed like a celebration for the butterfly's freedom. This early lesson in kindness stayed with me.

Several years later, our family went on summer vacation in the countryside of South-Western France at Lac (Lake) de Lacanau, close to Bordeaux. We had a great few weeks there, riding bikes through the woods, and my dad taught me how to swim. On our drive back to Paris, we were involved in a multi-car accident. The side of our car was badly damaged and could no longer be driven. Fortunately, no one was hurt.

We still had to get to Paris, rent a car and get back to Germany. My parents didn't speak French and, there in the French countryside, we had a hard time finding people to speak with us in German or English, and this made things even more difficult and stressful.

Finally, after two days, we were sitting in the rental car in the Paris traffic. My dad was still shaken from the accident and ordeal and wasn't used to the French way of driving. We were lost and didn't have a map.

Then a small miracle happened. At a stoplight, my mum, sitting in the back with me, cranked the window down and expressed to pedestrians that we needed help. One man spoke English, and he immediately understood our plight. He checked my father's eyes for permission, jumped into the passenger seat, guided us through Paris to the highway and at the last minute got out, waving after us. My parents were blown away.

From then on, I knew that small, miraculous moments can occur. I felt like the butterfly who had just been freed. Now, whenever I have the chance, I try to find those opportunities to be kind and assist someone, just as I did for the butterfly with my grandma, and that amazing stranger did for us on the streets of Paris so long ago.

"Share your good with others. Kindness, love and appreciation are the greatest gifts you can give."

—Louise Hay

The Day I Met Lori
By Beverly Shankman

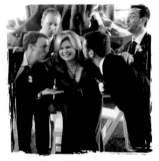

If Lori hadn't been there when I died, I would have stood with my parents in heaven and watched as someone else had the honor of walking each of my four sons down the aisle this year and giving them away to their brides.

If Lori hadn't been there when I died, the toasts I made before each wedding—telling my sons and their brides how much I love them, how proud I am of them, how excited I am that they found each other and how eagerly I anticipate the next step on their journeys—would have been left unsaid.

Because Lori was there when I died, I was alive to celebrate with my sons and future daughters-in-law as each of the four couples were engaged. Each time we received the call to let us know, "She said yes!" I looked up to the heavens in gratitude for yet another blessing and the knowledge that I had come very close to missing this joy.

If Lori hadn't been there when I died so much would have been left unsaid, undone and unexpressed. So many relationships would have never begun. So many people would not have been met. So much love would not have grown to depths so far beyond what it was before.

So please bear with me while I tell you the story of the day I met Lori.

My husband, Paul, and I did not know that morning was any different from any other Saturday morning or that it would change our lives forever. We got up as usual, enjoyed a cup of coffee together and left the house separately. He was going to the golf driving range. I was meeting a friend at yoga and going with her to lunch.

It had been a heartbreaking week. I had returned Monday from visiting my kids in LA. On the flight, I watched for hours as the news stations followed the story of the Boston Marathon bombing. When I got off the plane, my phone rang. A family member was calling to tell me my cousin had died two hours earlier—a cousin I loved deeply, who had been there whenever the boys or I needed him. I didn't know at the time that I would visit with him in heaven a few days later.

I got out of my car at 10:13, walked into the studio and greeted my friend. Handing her a little homemade gift, I registered for the class and stepped away to hang up my jacket.

I never made the five feet to the coat hook. Instead, my heart stopped. My head hit the registration desk, and I fell to the floor. No pulse. No breathing.

Erin, a yoga teacher, started resuscitation. Mary called 911 and had the paramedics on the phone as they told her how to start CPR. My friend stood shocked. She still apologizes, saying, "I just stood there. I didn't know what to do!" Another friend was trapped in the bathroom because my body was blocking the door.

Lori got out of her car at 10:16. Lori lives in Chicago, 350 miles away. She is a nurse with thirty-five years of emergency room and surgery experience. She was visiting the yoga studio as a space in which to see her Cleveland-based Ki-Hara (strengthening and resistance training) clients. She had not been there for several months, and we had never met. My explanation now for her presence is that my time wasn't up; God sent an angel to save my life.

Lori walked into the studio and saw me on the floor. She dropped her bags and fell to her knees to begin CPR. She tells me she brought me back for a moment—I opened my eyes and mumbled something—and then she lost me again. She brought me back once more and kept me oxygenated and pink until the paramedics came in with the paddles, which they used three times on the spot.

Lori told me later that she doesn't take full credit for my broken sternum and ribs. "Those paramedics were pretty big guys," she says. I still blame her. It took a broken sternum to save my life, and Lori to break it.

I refer to that day as "the day I met Lori," but I didn't actually become aware of her presence until the next day when she and the owner of the yoga studio visited me in the CICU at the Cleveland Clinic.

I spent a week in the hospital and left with a diagnosis of Takotsubo cardiomyopathy (broken-heart syndrome) and a brand-new internal automatic defibrillator, just in case it ever happens again (a one in a million chance). I was told I had the heart health of a ten-year-old boy: no blockages, no structural problems or damage. Just the hormonal effect on my heart of too much sadness. It was "broken."

My dad had died. Eight months later, Mom died. Five months after that, Paul's mom died. And then my cousin died. My heart was "broken," so it stopped. And my quest and journey began.

I met Lori for a Ki-Hara session a few weeks later. We agreed to work only on my lower body, because my sternum and ribs would not be healed for another year or so. I was able to walk eight steps at first. Then I managed sixteen. Motivated to stand in a river, craving to be near moving water, I walked thirty-two steps, and actually stopped to hug a tree as I caught my breath, and then walked thirty-two more with Paul. My cousin's widow held my arm as we walked slowly around the cul-de-sac. Once so simple; now a walk I could not manage on my own.

As I recovered, Lori and I met for coffee, walks and more Ki-Hara work when she came to town. During one of our visits a few months later she told me, "I am putting together a team to do the Hancock Tower stair climb in February."

"That's great!" I told her. "How many people will be on your team?"

"Including you, eight."

I laughed. I knew she was kidding.

She wasn't.

"Lori," I said. "Remember me? I'm the person whose life you just saved. I just had a cardiac arrest. You can't be serious."

"Oh, I'm serious," she replied in her assertive trainer's voice. "It's time for you to get up and get going again. First, you need to get permission from your cardiologist. Then we are going to take it slow. We'll start training now, work up to it, and in February you will be climbing the Hancock Tower with the team."

I got permission from my physician, Dr. Michael Faulx, who told me, "Climb the Hancock? Well, that's not a normal request, but if you want to, who am I to stop you?"

So I trained and trained some more, and then I climbed. I admit to being reassured that right behind me on the stairs at the climb were five paramedics. They told me they had my back. We huffed and puffed together to the top of that tower. Paul waited with water and hugs; my son and his girlfriend (now daughter-in-law!) were waiting with celebratory flowers.

Lori is no longer a stranger. She comes to Cleveland every two or three weeks to take care of her Ki-Hara clients, and we get together most times. I'm sure I mention each time just how we met, and twice we have hugged on the spot where it all happened. But now Lori is my friend. She is important in so many ways because if Lori hadn't been there when I died,

I am pretty sure I would have been a statistic. Nine out of ten sudden cardiac arrests that occur outside the hospital are fatal. But Lori was there. And because this stranger stopped to save a life, I am here to tell the story. Because a stranger stopped to save my life, I am making it my life's work to help others save their own and have gone on to become a yoga instructor and obtained a degree in holistic healing and, I hope my story has inspired you to consider a course in CPR.

The American Red Cross offers numerous classes online and in the classroom, so you can learn first aid, CPR, lifeguarding, babysitting, child care, swimming, family safety, water safety and more. The American Heart Association is another good source for online and classroom training. A few hours investment could save the life of someone dear to you or a stranger.

Loving Kindness Meditation

You've arrived. You're almost through the "kind stranger" stories. Whether it took you an hour, a day, a week, or a year to get this spot, it's of no matter. What matters is that you have arrived and that you're continuing to learn about the struggles others have been through and the ways these challenges have been lessened thanks to the kindness of strangers. Hopefully, by reading the stories, you have begun to observe openings in your environment to see someone in need and are inspired to seize the moment and act in a kinder fashion toward them. As you are learning from the stories, there are countless ways of being kind.

Perhaps you would like to choose this moment to learn a new way of being kind to yourself and add another way to expand your consciousness about kindness. It's called Loving Kindness Meditation (LKM). The process is very simple. By incorporating LKM into your life, you train your brain to focus on cultivating even more kindness while reaping the rewards of deep relaxation.

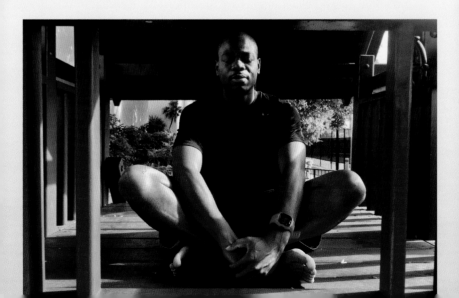

Begin by sitting or lying in a comfortable position, preferably in a quiet location. Turn your attention toward your breath, and take three to five slow, deep inhalations and long exhalations. Remember that when you exhale, you stimulate your vagus nerve and your heart rate slows.

Bring your attention to your heart, and say out loud or in your head, "May I be well. May I be happy. May I be at ease."

Next, think of someone you love or care about. You can mention them by name or group, or simply reflect on them. Say out loud or in your head, "May you or 'X' be well. May you or 'X' be happy. May you or 'X' be at ease."

Repeat this cycle for loved ones, friends, colleagues and acquaintances. You may choose to widen the circle to include even people you have never met or ones you don't get along with.

You can repeat this cycle, and continue widening the circle until you are wishing wellbeing, happiness and ease for the whole world. You can also choose to focus just on yourself and those closest to you. There are no rights or wrongs in LKM. The process is designed to help you reach a place of relaxation and comfort, and exact details are unimportant. Remain in this state for five to twenty minutes, and then gently emerge, and continue with your day.

By incorporating this meditation, or any form of deep relaxation, you are being kinder to yourself. We live in a fast-paced, stressful world, and we owe ourselves these moments of rest, reflection and contemplation.

Sailing Lessons
By Michael Thoennes

A few summers ago, I had the rare privilege of teaching a blind man to sail. For four years, I had worked at an aquatic sailing center teaching students aged eight to seventy-six, with varying disabilities such as cerebral palsy, autism and Down's syndrome. These experiences helped to shape me, and I am forever grateful for all the lessons I learned.

Although I have enjoyed all of it, nothing compared to teaching one sightless student to sail. No matter how much he learned that day, I am certain that I learned far more. I taught him to hold a straight course in the busiest part of Biscayne Bay, and he taught me that anything is possible.

The day was particularly beautiful, with bright blue skies, white puffy clouds and winds of twelve knots. It all seemed perfect to me, and I was struck by the fact that my student could see none of it. As I wondered how he felt during our sail, I reflected back to my adventure in the Grand Bazaar of Istanbul, Turkey, the previous summer. Walking through the seemingly endless halls of the ancient marketplace, I was surrounded by thousands of people. The sights were so bright, I felt blinded. Heat was radiating off all the visitors who had come from far and wide to eat and shop. Vibrant smells from the various spices and food products filled the air. My taste buds were stinging from the bitter Turkish coffee, and my ears were ringing as they tried to catch the few words I understood. Those moments in the bazaar, with all my senses actively engaged, were very special. Lifelong memories were etched.

Was this the way my blind student felt? Did he feel more alive and engaged than the other students because his perceptions were enhanced by his other senses? Instead of seeing less, was he in fact appreciating more? Was his experience similar to how I had felt wandering through the crowded marketplace in Turkey? I imagined he sat on the boat and felt the warm sun caress his body, the wind wrap around his face. He tasted the cool, salty water as he listened intently to my instructions. He felt the boat rock every time he turned the wooden tiller, and he quickly learned to maintain a straight course. This special day on Biscayne Bay helped me understand how to overcome adversity by adapting and utilizing other sensations to chart a course. It taught me to stay present in the moment, to take chances and not be impeded by perceptions of what is or is not possible.

I felt proud instructing a blind man to sail.

> "It's a little embarrassing after 45 years of research and study, the best advice I can give people is to be a little kinder to each other."
>
> —Aldous Huxley

Miracle Messages
By Jennifer Gottshall-Gavitt

I grew up in a town called Montoursville in Pennsylvania. It was a tight-knit community where everyone knew everyone else. Our grandfather was the Chief of Police. I still live nearby in a town that is even smaller. This story is about the incredible kindness of my small town and the way we look out for one another, even in the face of very difficult family times.

I had last seen my brother, Jeff, in 1996. He was twenty-seven and had been working at a construction company. He came home for a week to visit our dad. One day he said he was going out for coffee and never came back.

In 2001, right after I got married, I received a letter from him in which he said he was in California. I wrote back, but he never answered. I thought the next time I would hear about him would be from the authorities, telling me that he was dead, and I would have to come claim the body.

On Christmas Eve, 2014, my husband, Mike, got a phone call that would change our lives. A man named Kevin Adler, in San Francisco, California, had decided to try to help homeless men and women find their families. He'd created a nonprofit called Miracle Messages and began making short videos and posting them to social media to help reunite families. My brother was the first man he recorded. My friend saw the video on Facebook and recognized my brother and called to tell me the news.

I watched the video and said, "That looks like my brother." Later that night I went on social media and made a statement that I had seen my brother and that I would keep people in the town updated. We received many offers of help that night.

I called Jeff on Christmas Day, and we talked. I then called the local police who have an outreach team and asked them to help me get him home. They told me my brother had a serious alcohol problem, and they didn't think he could make it here without drinking. I didn't want to bring him home if I couldn't get him into rehab. How could I get him medical help? A state agency told me to bring him home and get him arrested because it would be easier to get him into treatment that way.

I called our Congressman and spoke to one of the aides. I told him what the agency had suggested and asked if the Congressman could help. The next day three facilities called and told me they had a bed. Then I called the assistance office and asked how to get insurance. They said he couldn't get insurance unless he had been a county resident for six months. But then the director of the county public assistance office called and said Jeff could have insurance immediately. He too had heard from the Congressman.

I went out to San Francisco to see Jeff at the end of June. We met for breakfast, and he was drinking at nine a.m.

I had done everything to get him to treatment, but he didn't want to come. He didn't want to be put in the system. I explored the option of having him involuntarily committed. Police officers said he was polite and not a danger to self or others, so I could not commit him.

Our story doesn't have the typical happy ending. But I am so much happier now that I have found my brother. He says he feels like the street is his home. He now knows that he can call me, and he does so at random times. He knows that people check up on him at my request. Members of the police outreach team will look after him and send me a message periodically.

Now he has people who know where he is, and I feel better because my brother isn't lost. When I can't sleep at night, I don't have to wonder where he is. My dad, who is 72, now has peace of mind knowing that one of his kids isn't lost somewhere. I can reassure my dad that Jeff is fine.

The entire town has had my back. That is so humbling and life-affirming. I had people messaging me with all kinds of support. Some told me, "When your brother comes home, I will give him a job." Others offered to go to California and bring him home. Others offered their car and a place to stay. I still get messages of concern and care. This has been the closest thing to a spiritual epiphany on earth.

"Do your little bit of good where you are; it's those little bits of good put together that overwhelm the world."

—Desmond Tutu

Tomas
By Layne Harris

I began working as the General Manager at the Café at Books & Books on Lincoln Road, a pedestrian mall in the heart of South Beach, Miami Beach, in 2014. I had no experience in hospitality but was excited to begin this new challenge in my life. The restaurant has many regular customers but none like Tomas.

Mirian, one of our waitresses, remembers the first day he came in. His lunch was $32, and he paid in cash. A few minutes later, he tried to pay again. Mirian was confused and alerted me.

Tomas began coming more often. The staff got to know him, and it became apparent that he had some memory issues. Even though he had only ordered minutes before, he would get impatient with waitstaff at times and ask, "Where is my food?" At first, the waitstaff felt he was being rude, but they quickly learned that they were dealing with a unique situation, and they were very compassionate with him. Instead of getting defensive and telling him he just ordered, they would gently say, "Let me go check."

Over time, we all grew fond of Tomas. As more time passed, he began eating all his meals at Books & Books. He always ordered the same thing: for breakfast it was eggs, for lunch a bowl of soup, a burger rare, no bun and a salad or crab cakes. Same order for dinner, and he always had a Diet Coke. He would eat the whole burger and always left the salad.

When we asked Tomas why he ordered the salad but didn't eat it, he said, "I like the way it looks on the plate." At the end of each meal, he would order a Cortadito (Cuban coffee with steamed milk) and we would make sure to give him decaf with skim milk, as we worried about his health. He informed the staff he was a diabetic, so when he asked for a dessert, we usually told him we had run out. About once a week, we would give him a dessert as a special treat. His favorite was the apple pie.

He always ordered grilled chicken, which he took home for his cat. We worried that this was an unnecessary expense for Tomas, so we bought cat food and portioned some out daily. Sometimes, he would just come by to pick up the cat food.

At times, Tomas would lose his wallet and wouldn't be able to pay. I was awed by the staff, each of whom took care of him even though it would cost them money. The waitstaff still had to tip out the bussers and food runners, so not only were they investing their time in taking care of a customer who didn't tip, but they were out of pocket. Yet no one complained.

We ended up creating a separate way of billing for him. We developed a special button on our point of sale system and called it the Tomas Comp. A credit card was kept on file and we used it. Tomas would always ask if we were being paid. That was a huge concern of his. No matter what, we all reassured him that he need not worry. We knew he needed to eat.

He shared with us that he was born in Havana and had become an actor to overcome his shyness. We read about him on the Internet and learned that he had come to the U.S. as a young man, had studied at the Actors Studio in New York, and become an American citizen. In 1958, he went to Italy to take part in the theater festival in Spoleto.

He decided to relocate to Italy and lived there for 25 years. He was a very handsome man in his earlier days. He was known as a "Spaghetti Western star" in the 1970s and became an Italian celebrity. He was also in many successful movies when he returned to the U.S., such as Amistad (1996) and Traffic (2000). He told us that he became very famous in Italy and had grown weary of being recognized everywhere he went. He returned to the U.S., where he was only recognized on occasion, and he found that to be more comfortable.

At one point, Tomas was coming to Books & Books up to six times a day. He would eat, then forget that he had just eaten and return and try to order again. The staff continued to keep an eye on him. If he'd just finished a big meal, they knew to order him soup. We knew this was the final chapter of his life, and we wanted to make it as happy as possible.

He lived a few blocks away and would walk here, then wander the streets and return. As time passed and his disease progressed, he became more docile and no longer criticized my staff. Eventually, he returned to the kind-hearted soul that he had always been. He was very appreciative of the attention and care he received and always expressed genuine gratitude. He told me there was a book written about him and although it was in Italian, I expressed interest in seeing it. Shortly after, Tomas brought it in and even signed it. He wrote, "To Layne" and then drew a heart with sunbursts coming out the sides. He signed his name, "Tomas." He was so proud and showed me some pictures of how he looked when he was a budding actor. So handsome and even a little gangster looking. Tomas said he was the complete opposite of his characters. I will forever cherish this book.

As the years passed, we all felt like a team helping Tomas. It was satisfying to see how we all shared a common goal of keeping him as happy and healthy as we could. He gave us a sense of purpose that can often be missing in our hurried world.

March 22, 2017, was a beautiful sunny day, like so many in Miami Beach. We waited for Tomas but he didn't show up. We tried and tried to reach him, but we had no luck. We didn't know where he lived, so we were at a loss as to what to do. After a few days, we got a message from a family member saying he had died of natural causes. He was 84 when he passed away. We are all so sad. We miss him.

The experience with Tomas changed each of us, which we each feel is his beautiful legacy. Our staff has bonded in a special way. Tomas allowed us to be the best versions of ourselves. We each saw one another contributing and it increased our desire to help and our respect for one another. And we have learned to be more tolerant of those with mental illness. We now have a new customer who has a different set of challenges. He comes in three times a day, and we are happy to accommodate his preferences the way we did for Tomas.

I am so happy that everyone came together to give what they could to make Tomas's last years happy. It was heartwarming to see everyone take in a stranger and care for him daily for three years. We miss him and are comforted by the fact that we were able to provide so much to him at the end of his long life.

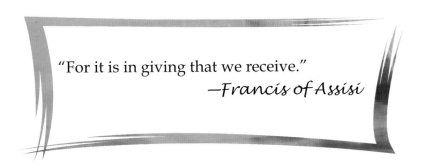

"For it is in giving that we receive."
—Francis of Assisi

Is Kindness Genetic?

Did you ever meet someone who just seems effortlessly kind? It's almost like their default mode. No matter where they go or what they are doing, they always seem to be helping someone. Perhaps you have a friend, relative, doctor, nurse or therapist you know who fits this description. Could kindness be in their genes? Maybe!

Aleksandr Kogan, Ph.D. at the University of Cambridge, along with his colleagues, showed that one-third of the population they studied had a specific combination of genes and they displayed "more prosocial behavior."

The late Paul Walker was a huge advocate of random acts of kindness and an expert at keeping it under the radar. In 2004, the famous actor anonymously bought an engagement ring for Iraq War veteran Kyle Upham and his fiancée, Kristin. The couple had been scouting out rings at a Santa Barbara, California, jewelry store but Upham couldn't afford his future bride's dream diamond, which was priced over $10,000. After overhearing the couple, Walker told the manager to put the ring on his tab and quietly walked out of the store.

The couple was completely floored by the unknown man's generosity, but when they asked who had paid for it, they were told by store staff that it was an anonymous gift. The sales clerk kept the story a secret until after Walker's death when she decided to go public with it; she wanted everyone to know what a remarkable person Walker had been.

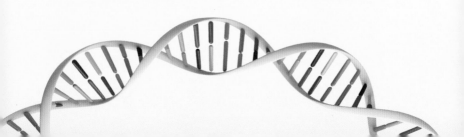

The Invisible Girl
By Katherine Magnoli

One day I was sitting in my wheelchair, rolling along vigorously to get to class on time. Just as I was about to turn the corner and go down the ramp, I noticed one of my shoes had fallen off. I picked it up, and lifted my leg onto the bench and began trying to place the shoe back on my foot. This sounds like a simple task, but it was nothing of the sort. You see, my chair had poor brakes and kept moving back and forth, and it was not easy to get the shoe back on.

As I struggled, I noticed a number of people glance in my direction but walk by as if I were invisible. Then, all of a sudden, a fellow student, whom I had never met, was kneeling before me. He asked if I needed help, and I laughed and said, "Yes, that would be great! I really need to get to class."

He replied, "Yes, I know. I can't believe no one offered you help before. That is really sad."

I nodded, and the boy gave me his number and said if I ever needed anything else to call him and he would always be able to help. I smiled, and I still smile every time I think of him. I haven't needed his help again, but what a comfort it is to know that there are good people nearby, always ready to lend a hand. Knowing this gives me the confidence to take risks and to lead a more adventurous, fulfilling and purposeful life.

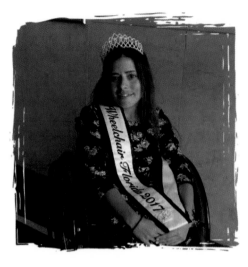

Postscript: Kat no longer feels invisible. After college, she continued her education and attended leadership and self-advocacy training programs. She is the co-host of an online radio show, a model for the Bold Beauty Project, publishes her own books called *The Adventures of KatGirl* and in April 2017, she was crowned Ms. Wheelchair Florida.

"For beautiful eyes, look for the good in others; for beautiful lips, speak only words of kindness; and for poise, walk with the knowledge that you are never alone."

—*Audrey Hepburn*

Who's Bob?
By Patrick Doval

I've been a musician for most of my life. My songs and albums have sold around the world, yet I have never been fortunate enough to get a record deal or been able to tour to support my albums. I had only performed in front of an audience a handful of times, although it was something I really loved to do. One day a former co-worker, Richard, told me about an open mic event at the Miami Beach Urban Studios at Florida International University hosted by Robert Zuckerman. I decided to go and give it a shot.

When I got to the studios I met the host and asked, "Are you Robert Zimmerman?" I'd gotten his name wrong! So much for making a good first impression. I apologized and told him I'd been thinking of Bob Dylan (whose real name is Robert Zimmerman). Robert opened up and began telling me about who he was and what he did. He was a Hollywood photographer, the real deal—a legend. His stories inspired me. I gained confidence from his encouragement and began to look forward to each open mic event. I began to write songs structured for the format. I changed my style to suit the space and to please Robert and the audience.

I gained self-confidence in performing and got better each month. Robert became my mentor and I am, without a doubt, a better human being and musician because of him. He recently gave me the opportunity to play music at his exhibit, where I met Khalilah Ali (the former Mrs. Muhammad Ali). What an honor!

Before I met Robert, I had forgotten I was a musician. I was on the verge of giving up something I dearly loved, but now I am a few weeks away from releasing a new album. Robert even took the photos! One of my songs will be sent to commercial and college radio stations across the country. I've found my voice and my life has new meaning, thanks to the support and encouragement of my friend Robert. What a difference one person can make.

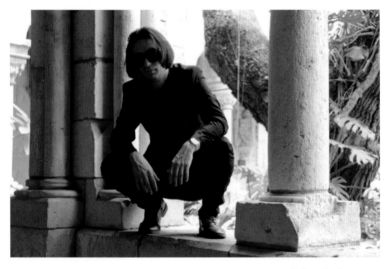

© Robert Zuckerman

"Service to others is the rent you pay for your room here on earth."

—Muhammad Ali

Set Free
By Eva Ritvo

Expectant parents often say, "I just want my child to be healthy." I too felt that way, but it wasn't to be the case. When my daughter, Joy, was five months old, she was diagnosed with a form of cerebral palsy known as hemiparesis, meaning weakness in half of her body. When she was two-and-a-half years old, she began having seizures. Needless to say, life has presented numerous challenges for Joy and for those of us who love her dearly.

Shortly after receiving Joy's diagnosis, one of my mentors shared his experience that, "A family is held hostage by its sickest member." Over the years, I found that to be true.

Joy's limitations came in many forms. She was late in walking and never developed the use of her left hand. Her seizures became life-threatening, and at age five, as a last resort, she underwent brain surgery. Thirty-six hours later, she stopped breathing and required a second emergency operation to bring her back to life. She never had another seizure, but she was left with a host of other problems. For the next several years life revolved around doctor and therapy visits. She required daily treatment for many years to maximize her ability to walk, talk and perform other tasks.

My life was impacted in myriad ways: constant anxiety, fear of being away from my daughter, learning to manage complicated medical issues, and so on. Despite being trained as a physician, I felt overwhelmed by the responsibility and the weight of the decisions that had to be made. My husband and I approached Joy's illnesses and treatments differently. Our marriage suffered and eventually ended. Joy's sister grew up fast; the three of us stuck close together. Many friends did not grasp the depth of Joy's disability and criticized me for being overprotective. Many withdrew.

Because of the very real possibility of a life threatening seizure, we were instructed to remain within ten minutes of an emergency room. Thus, air travel was strictly prohibited. My nearest family members lived 1,000 miles away and the isolation took a toll.

Years passed, life slowly improved, and with a lot of support and hard work, Joy was able to finish high school. The transition to college was very rocky and it often felt as though we would remain by one another's side indefinitely. I worried about my health and how Joy would survive should something happen to me.

In 2014, my dear friend, Rochelle Baer, and I co-founded the Bold Beauty Project (BBP), a nonprofit that pairs women with disabilities with award-winning photographers to create art exhibits showcasing the beauty of these extraordinary women. To my wonderment and relief, our family began to experience a reversal of fortune. Since then, I have come to learn that the inverse of the parable is also true. When the sickest member heals, so, too, does the rest of the family. Our healer came from the art world, a world that Joy has always found to be the most therapeutic.

When Rochelle was looking for a venue for our next show, she was given the name of a photography professor, Robert Zuckerman. I looked Robert up and discovered that he was quite a force of nature—a brilliant and highly regarded man who had founded or was active on behalf of multiple charities. Will Smith called him "the Picasso of photography." What I didn't read online were the challenges that Robert had faced in his own life: his mother and sister were disabled, and he was wheelchair-bound due to a progressive illness.

We connected by email, and I told Robert about our project. He was very receptive, so I invited him to lunch to discuss his possible participation. Shortly after the food arrived, I asked him if he would photograph Joy. (You know how moms are— when it comes to helping our kids, we can be pretty gutsy!) He said "yes" and thus began the process of freeing our family.

Robert visited our home a week later with an entourage. He brought a seven-year-old "assistant," a boy battling leukemia who dreamed of becoming a photographer. Robert decided to make his dream a reality, and the boy has been assisting Robert ever since. He also brought his assistant's mother and a beautiful young woman named Zoraida, who is hearing impaired. Zoraida was excited to become a Bold Beauty model.

Joy was skeptical at first but quickly warmed to Robert and his group. I sensed something special was happening, so I stayed out of the way and let the magic happen. It wasn't long before Joy looked and felt beautiful in front of the camera. When Robert surprised her by asking her if she wanted to photograph Zoraida, Joy was over the moon. Joy often feels that she is on the sidelines of life, watching others enjoy things she cannot. But on that day, she was front and center. It was glorious.

Joy had chosen to be photographed amongst red rose petals. At one point, Robert had Zoraida rain them down on her. Joy seemed to transition from a shy girl to a confident women right before everyone's eyes.

Robert called the day a "love fest."

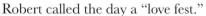

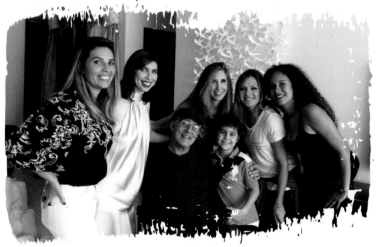

Robert continued to work with Joy, and they created
spectacular images that have been shown at international art
fairs attended by thousands of people and used on all the BBP
material. We keep two of them in the entryway of our home as
a constant source of Joy and inspiration. A third hangs in my
office.

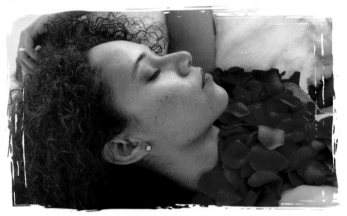

Zoraida Miller photographed by Joy Nestor and Robert Zuckerman

Joy's confidence has soared, and she has been gradually
gaining her independence. Robert continues to support and
encourage her at art shows and via Facebook and texts, and
his affection has been transformative. When asked how he feels
about their relationship, Robert replied, "It literally brings me
Joy."

Joy sees how Robert's disability doesn't slow him down, and
he shared that his situation has heightened his compassion
for others. He gave up the most glamorous of lives, shooting
Hollywood celebrities, and can now be found photographing
children at the local hospitals, running a nonprofit he co-
founded, Hope and Carry (teaching inner city kids to shoot
with cameras instead of guns), coordinating his World
Betterment Symposium, or helping Joy, or the many other
people he has taken under his wing like Patrick, in the
proceeding story. He seems to be an insatiable giver!

Robert has provided Joy with a positive role model. As a result, she is taking more risks as she feels her safety net has broadened. She is now living in a dorm 45 minutes from home and has gained the confidence to go places on her own. Thanks to the support of excellent tutors, she is doing well academically. She is engaging more with friends, and (spoiler alert) she has fallen in love as you will read about in the next and final story.

It feels like a miracle to watch her grow, enjoying life in a way she previously hadn't. Joy's sister, Gigi, is thriving in college, far from home. The heightened sense of responsibility gained from her childhood has served her well.

In our own ways, we have each indeed been set free.

I deeply appreciate the opportunity to work on the Bold Beauty Project. I am so grateful to have found time to create this book and to share what Joy, Robert and others have taught me about the power of kindness, the ability to see beauty in so many more places, and the possibilities we all have to transcend our limitations and live with greater freedom.

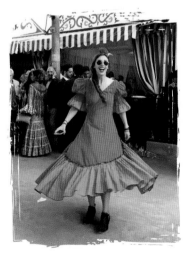

Gigi in Seville, Spain

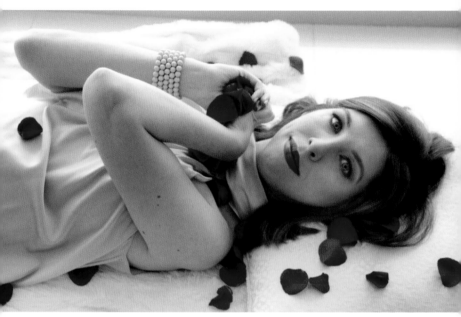

Joy photographed for the Bold Beauty Project
© Robert Zuckerman

"The highest purpose of art is to inspire.
What else can you do? What else can
you do for anyone but inspire them."
—Bob Dylan

My Fairy Tale Come True
By Joy Nestor

Almost every little girl dreams about living a fairy tale life and meeting a prince and falling in love, but not all find it. I'm one of the lucky few that did get her prince. Don't get the wrong idea, my Vince isn't a traditional, son-of-a-king type of prince, he's an even rarer type of prince—he's one because of his kindness, generosity and love. And as far as I'm concerned, that's the best type of prince a girl can have!

Just like all fairy tales, I've been through my share of trials and tribulations, as has my prince. About five months after my life-changing photo shoot with Robert Zuckerman, I decided I was tired of being lonely and wanted to find a boyfriend. Since I am shy, I decided going online would be my best option. I had tried online dating before and nothing good had come of it, but this time around I was determined. I knew what I was looking for, and I wasn't going to give up until I found it.

I decided to exercise my artistic license and wrote the most creative, catchy, and direct profile I could, and it worked! I weeded through the messages I received and chose a handful of guys who looked nice and cute (let's be real—I'm in my early 20's—cuteness does count!) to respond to. All of the guys started the text conversation with the typical formalities of questions, such as, "What's your favorite color?" except Vincent. With Vince, we almost immediately delved into deep and long conversations. Most of our messages to each other were long paragraphs, discussing anything and everything. Every day for three weeks, we would text from morning until night. I felt like I'd known him my whole life, and I hadn't even met him yet.

Our first date was really the beginning of our love story.

I didn't know it at the time, but he took a bus, got off at the wrong stop, and walked hours in the heat to meet me. I had been sick in bed all day with a migraine. None of that seemed to matter once he arrived. We gelled from the moment we met and became an official couple by the end of the day. I remember thinking that night as I fell asleep, I hope we are in love by the time our six-month anniversary rolls around. I'll let you in on a secret, it took a lot less time than that.

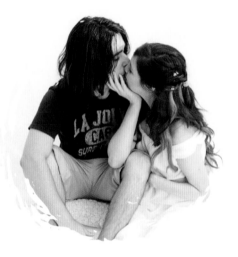

Vince was the piece of me that I never knew I was missing. I know it sounds cliché, but we really do complete each other. I swear sometimes he knows me better that I know myself. For example, he can tell when I'm getting too frustrated while trying to do something, and without even exchanging a word he'll help. Tasks I can do on my own he'll let me, and I can see him beaming with pride.

We know each other so well, that we can have conversations just by exchanging glances. Every moment I'm with him, (except for the ones when I have to kiss him goodbye) is the new best moment of my life. We don't need anything special to enjoy each other's company. Most of our favorite dates are the ones we spend cuddling, watching anime, or playing Pokémon on my DS.

We laugh. A lot. I think laughter is one of the best gifts a person can give, and I love that we share so much laughter together.

I'm a stronger, more confident person because he is in my life. We just celebrated our one year anniversary. I can already tell you, I can't wait to spend the rest of my life with him. We may have started off as strangers, but with the kindness, and love between us…he's become the love of my life.

My fairy tale is just getting started, and I can't wait to see where our story takes us!

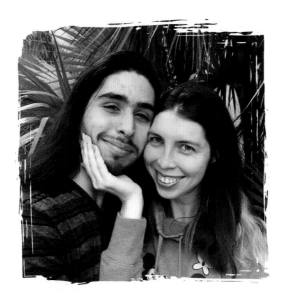

"Kindness is a free currency from a well that will never dry up."

—Lady Gaga

Afterword

Thank you for getting to this place in *Bekindr*. I hope you have been touched by the wide range of stories about kindness and that you have used this time as an opportunity to reflect on your own life. Who has been kind to you? To whom have you been kind? What sorts of impressions have these experiences left with you? How have they impacted your relationships? How can you Bekindr? I hope you have gained a broader perspective from which to draw your answers.

Have you learned to see more opportunities to Bekindr as you have been reading and reflecting on this topic? Have you lifted your nose out of your cell phone long enough to notice the person in front of you who might be struggling with the door or having a difficult day? You needn't look far to find a chance to help. Life is always presenting us with challenges, and kindness can smooth the edges. Slow down and let the driver next to you come into your lane. Honor pedestrians in crosswalks. Smile! So simple, but you can make someone's day and lower your own heart rate and blood pressure in the process.

As you put this book down, it's important that you don't lose focus. Distractions are everywhere. Being kind requires commitment; it's a practice, just like anything else. On the next page, you will find a few suggestions to help you remember to Bekindr. This book is about kindness to strangers, but I hope you'll always be kind to yourself first so that you are living your optimal life. When we thrive, it is so much easier to give to those around us. So please, take good care of yourself!

Take the *Bekindr* Challenge

Habit change isn't easy. Small changes can lead to big changes, so that's where we suggest you start. Make a commitment to adding a minimum of one minute of kindness to your day. Who doesn't have one minute to try to make their life and the lives of those around them better?

Start by placing two sticky notes on the mirror where you brush your teeth. If you travel a lot, tape the note to your toothpaste. One note should say "Bekindr today." The other note should say "What did I do to Bekindr today?"

It's that simple.

By focusing on kindness twice daily, you will find it easier to incorporate acts of kindness into your life. And when you do, you will feel happier and more connected to those around you. Refer back to the long list of ways to Bekindr. If you are very pressed for time, simply smile at someone. If you have more time, there are plenty of options to try out.

Try it for a few days or more and let us know it goes. We are eager to hear your stories at <u>Bekindr.com</u> and on Facebook!

Take the Kindness Quiz:

On Bekindr.com, you can find quizzes to help you assess your current level of kindness. Retake them after a month and see if there has been any change in your score. And don't worry, no one is grading them! They are there simply to help you focus on the presence of kindness in your life

Acknowledgments

The inspiration for this book emerged out of a transformative experience with a kind stranger, Louie B. Free. Louie, I am forever grateful. Patrice Samara, thank you for believing in the project and bringing *Bekindr* to life. Ian Halperin and Katie Arnold-Ratliff, thank you for sorting through and editing hundreds of stories. That was a huge task and I am very appreciative. Emily Jarecki, Jean Krag, Nick and Diane Marson, Tracy Masington, Joy Nestor, Pamela Page, Liliana and Jose Retelny, Ed & Matt Ritvo, Shomberg Ulysse and Allan Varah: thanks for all your writing and editing assistance. To my sister, Deborah Louria, I can't thank you enough for all you did to improve this book. You dropped everything to assist and I am so grateful for your expertise and your kindness. Thank you to my other sister, Anne Bielamowicz, for sharing your story and your photography in addition to editorial assistance. Jessica Kizorek, thank you for the headshot and for making me look and BE my best!

To my daughters, Joy and Gigi thank you for *everything*!

Anthony Liggins, thank you for your friendship and constant encouragement and for providing artistic oversight and sharing your art with *Bekindr* and the world. Robert Zuckerman, I could not have done it without you! Thank you for sharing your huge heart, your story and beautiful photography. Pablo Fenjves and Daniel Gilfarb, you planted the seeds for this project and your kindness throughout the project is greatly appreciated. Craig Calvert, thank you for all your assistance along this path. Adeline Oka and Daniel Passman, thank you for providing crucial support to *Bekindr*. Judith Regan and Emily Greenwald, Martin Rouillard thank you for all you have done to nurture *Bekindr*. Lorena Fernandez, Donelle Dunstall and the Elite Flyers team, and Momosa Publishing team, thank you for bringing the project home!

Thank you to Frank Fiorello and Richard Winkler from *Come From Away*. Meeting Nick and Diane and seeing your show has been one of the highlights of the project. Thank you to Layne Harris, David and all the staff at Books & Books for your support along the way.

Like all complex projects, it takes a village. Thank you as well to all the following who participated: Dhardra Blake, Lisa Bloch, Marilyn Caiola, Castellanos family, Dara and Lior Cohen, Léna Cohen, Mariana Cruz, Susan Fleming, Julio Flores, Raymond Fornino, Valeria Geritzen, Ira Glick, Caren and Andy Glickson, Kerry Gruson, Jennifer Hoberman, Robert Holmes, David and Lee Ann Lester, Eli Levy, Adam and Lizeth Lowe, Debra Luftman, the Masington family, including Hanoch and Beverly McCarty, Barbara Mason, Renu Moody, Adrian Muller, Terry Newmyer, Michael Noltemeyer, Vincent Peloso, Robert Polishook, Gonzalo Quesada, Tom Rodman, Suzie Salowe, Meital Stavinsky, Jimena Stein, Tatjana Terzic, Osamu Toki, Tim Vandehey, Neelam Varshney, Catrine Washington and Eros Yabut and so many others.

I am so grateful to all those who have shown and taught me about kindness: my parents, siblings, children, friends, colleagues, patients, and strangers. Kindness is indeed everywhere.

Thank you to each of you who shared your story with us. This project is a reflection of all your efforts, and I have enjoyed getting to know each one of you and learning from you. My only regret is that all 220 stories that were submitted could not be included in this book.

And last but not least, thank you, the reader for sharing your valuable time and interest. I am wishing you a life filled with kindness.

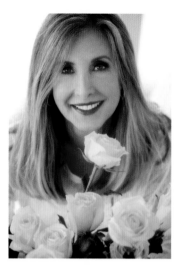

Eva Ritvo, MD is a psychiatrist with over twenty-five years of experience practicing in Miami Beach, Florida. She is the founder of Bekindr®, a movement to foster more kindness in the world. She is also the co-founder of the Bold Beauty Project (BBP), a nonprofit that pairs women with disabilities with award-winning photographers and creates art shows. BBP is dedicated to breaking stereotypes and raising awareness about the beauty to be found in all women including those with disabilities.

Dr. Ritvo is the former Chair of Psychiatry and Behavioral Medicine at Mount Sinai Medical Center and the former Vice Chair of Psychiatry and Behavioral Sciences at the Miller School of Medicine at the University of Miami. She is a Distinguished Fellow of the American Psychiatry Association and a member of the American College of Psychiatrists.

She is on the board of United Cerebral Palsy Foundation, which was recently renamed United Community Options. In 2015, she was recognized as their National Volunteer of the Year.

Dr. Ritvo received her undergraduate and medical degrees from UCLA and completed her psychiatry residency training at Weill Cornell Medicine. She is the mother of two adult daughters.